Order this book and study guide from:
All Nations Publications
P.O. Box 92847
Southlake, Texas 76092
1-817-514-0653

ISBN: 0-9662085-5-2

***Other Books by Roger Sapp available from
All Nations Publications:***

The Last Apostles on Earth, *A popular textbook on apostles and apostolic ministry. Sold in 20 countries the first year of publication. 186 pages, 1995*
Pandora's Pulpit, *A Biblical study that supports women in ministry and encourages New Testament apostolic government in the Church. Particularly reveals the prophetess in Scripture. 250 pages, 1998*
Apostolic Fathers and Spiritual Bastards, *A Biblical Review of the Essential Ministry Father Doctrine, a popular and abusive heresy. 110 pages, 1999*

Performing Miracles and Healing

A Biblical Guide to Developing a Christ-like Supernatural Ministry

Roger Sapp

Printed in the United States by:
Morris Publishing
3212 East Highway 30
Kearney, NE 68847
1-800-650-7888

Acknowledgements

If there is any merit to the book that you are holding, it is due almost entirely to the patience of Jesus Christ. He teaches ordinary people how to do extraordinary things. I want to thank many others as well for their assistance. My wife and best friend, Ann, again endured through my writing another book. She again tirelessly read various drafts of this book and commented insightfully.

Various pastors were helpful without knowing it. As Christ healed the sick and injured at their churches, some pastors asked me important practical questions about how this works. They enabled me to discover more areas of theological concerns and misunderstandings that I had overlooked.

My father, Nelson Sapp, was also helpful in asking me some difficult questions after he read the initial draft of the book. I responded to his questions in various sections of the book.

Sue Fincher, who edited one of my previous books, also edited this book. Sue has an incredible mix of gifts, skills, and experience. She offered me a great deal of wisdom in presentation and precision of message as she did in the previous book.

Finally, I would like to thank the all the believers at Restoration Church in Euless, Texas, particularly Pastor C. Douglas White and the elders and staff for being my friends and an extended family to us.

Contents

Foreword

Roger Sapp has provided all believers, but especially those of us in Christian ministry, with an invaluable tool. This book will prove to be a great resource and encouragement to those who long to understand and apply the message of healing. We will all profit from the countless hours of thorough research Roger has given to this study. He has gathered all the accounts of healing in the New Testament and organized them in a way that is easy to comprehend and assimilate. As I read through the material I came to a renewed appreciation for the vast amount of scripture given to this subject. Healing is not treated as a side issue in God's Word. Our Lord spent a large amount of time healing people. What Roger has done is organize the biblical evidence about healing and present it in such a way that we are immediately challenged to reevaluate our personal attitude toward healing over against the scriptural record.

I must frankly admit that my own journey toward understanding healing has been, at times, full of uncertainty, confusion, fear and false assumptions. What I knew about healing was prejudiced by my cultural, denominational bias. What I didn't know about healing was hidden because of my unwillingness to honestly examine all the evidence continued in scripture related to healing. As a result of a personal "time of refreshing" from the Lord my heart was quickened to walk in obedience to Christ in all the areas of my life and ministry. While I prayed and waited before the Lord I heard Him say,

"You can believe what men say about My Word or you can believe My Word."

It was at this point, that I realized how dependent I had become on the opinions, interpretations, and attitudes of others. This realization rekindled a fire in me to study for myself what God had to say about healing, gifts, the Word of God, the Holy Spirit, etc. That is why I appreciate Roger's efforts so much. His focus on the original records can't help but better prepare us for service.

The emphasis that Roger gives to Christ and His healing ministry is profoundly important. He calls us again to a Christocentric attitude toward healing. Who do we want to be our model? Who are we to follow? The author challenges us to establish our ministry of healing on the foundation of Christ and Christ alone. As Jesus revealed the Father's heart to heal, so we are called to follow hard after His example.

If this book is radical, it is radical in a welcome way. It keeps reminding us of our spiritual heritage. We are always and forever to be a healing community.

This is not a book which attempts to answer all the questions we have about suffering and sickness. (Though many questions are answered at the conclusion of his work.) It is a book which casts unbelief aside and calls for a proactive faith to minister faithfully God's power and love to those who need healing.

We need to hear again the word given in James 5:13-15:

"Is anyone among you suffering? Let him pray. Is anyone cheerful? Let him sing praises. Is anyone among you sick? Let him call for the elders of the church, and let them pray over him, anointing him with oil in the name of the Lord; and the prayer offered in faith will restore the one who is sick, and the Lord will raise him up, and if he has committed sins, they will be forgiven him."

Read this book, study this book, then seek to boldly apply the revelation you receive. If you do, then there is no doubt that you will be blessed and even better, those you serve who are waiting for a touch from Christ through you will be blessed.

C. Douglas White
Senior Pastor, Restoration Church
Euless, Texas

Introduction

In the winter months of 1972, I received Christ as my Savior, Lord and Baptizer in the Holy Spirit. I can honestly say that I believed in divine healing from the beginning of my walk with Christ, and even had a number of personal healings and a few creative miracles of my own in my developing relationship with Christ in the two decades leading up to 1992. Reflecting back, I can see now that my theology of healing was very complex and impractical. I also occasionally suffered from sickness, and healing did not always seem available. My experience of healing during those two decades seemed mysterious, generally unreliable and unpredictable. This was true of my own personal experience as well as my prayer for others.

In 1992, I had a personal breakthrough in healing that transformed my thinking on this matter. In the Summer of 1992, while praying about another matter, the Spirit of Christ unexpectedly said this to me:

Why don't you receive Me as your Healer in the same way that you received Me as your Savior?

By asking me this simple question, Christ initiated in me a series of events and a renewed interest in what Scripture said on this matter. I began to meditate on Scripture and came to new conclusions on healing. I began to discover that my healing theology of twenty years was not really based on Scripture, but on my erratic healing experiences and what others had taught from their erratic experiences. Because my experiences had matched theirs, I accepted much of what I heard as being the truth, without serious examination and comparison with Scripture.

Because my experience of healing was unpredictable, unreliable and often seemed mysterious, I had adopted a popular modern healing theology that reflected that experience. However, I was still unaware that I had accepted many aspects of unbelieving philosophy on these matters that are common in our culture and in the Church in America.

I had socially acceptable, but scripturally wrong explanations for why healing did not occur. Inwardly, I knew there was something wrong with my experience. However, my intellectual explanations of healing, or why God did not heal, certainly matched my experience.

As I began to examine my beliefs on this matter in 1992, I could not reconcile what I then believed with Scripture. What was most apparent was that my beliefs were not in harmony with what Christ demonstrated and said about healing. I came to realize that my previous theology of healing didn't focus on Christ's example and teaching, but somehow had set Him aside as a *special example*, one that could not instruct me.

Because of this, my theology of healing relied heavily upon the Old Testament and a few New Testament verses regarding the lives of the followers of Christ.

Subsequently, I knew more about Paul's thorn in the flesh and Job's sufferings than I knew about the many detailed Gospel accounts of healings and miracles in Christ's ministry. I knew more of the common explanations for the value of suffering than I knew of Christ's words to the suffering people He encountered.

However, Christ did not allow me to continue in that mindset. In a matter of a few months, not only was my theology of healing transformed, but my experience as well. First, I was completely healed of a thirty-year chronic problem with sinus infections and the blinding headaches they caused. Secondly, because of being encouraged by my experience of healing, my wife Ann experienced healing of frequent migraine headaches which would last two or three days. She was also healed of severe asthma which required serious daily medication. My family's overall health also improved dramatically. All of us, in that season, experienced a reduction of suffering from illness and pain.

In a matter of a couple years, I began to see healing and creative miracles on a much greater scale in my public ministry. In some situations in my traveling ministry to local churches today as many as 75%-80% of the people attending are healed of some sort of condition. Many of the healings are visible to the congregations. Normally, in these kinds of meetings, I begin by showing Christ's willingness to heal by praying for people with injured and painful bad backs. Most often, all are visibly healed and are then able to bend without pain for the first time in a long time. When others there see this, that normally releases faith for healing of physical conditions that are not necessarily visible. Some of these healings are of minor conditions simply causing discomfort. Some healings are of very serious conditions which are extremely painful and often life threatening.

While the Lord grants healings as I travel today, the main focus of my ministry today is not healing the sick, but is rather equipping others to heal the sick. This is the purpose of this book. I am convinced that some who practice the *five-fold ministry* mentioned in Ephesians 4,[1] simply exercise their *gifts* but fail to exercise their *ministries*. The five-fold ministry is *to equip the saints for the work of ministry*.[2] In other words, every gifted minister ought to be teaching, discipling and leading others into the experience of ministry rather than just demonstrating their gifts.

If a minister knows how to heal the sick, then that minister ought to be teaching the people of God how to do this. If he knows how to cast out demons, then he should be teaching others how to do this rather than just doing it himself. If a prophet knows how to accurately prophesy, he should be teaching the people of God how to accurately prophesy. Likewise, the evangelist should be teaching others how to evangelize rather than just doing the work of evangelism himself. Therefore, this book is focused on releasing believers into the ministries of healing the sick and performing miracles. My hope is that readers of this

---

[1] The apostle Paul in Ephesians 4:11 lists five gift ministries. They are apostles, prophets, evangelists, pastors and teachers.
[2] Ephesians 4:12

book will excel in helping the suffering find healing and therefore glorify Christ by doing *His greater works*.[3]

The end of the age draws near. The Church must come to maturity in all matters and complete the harvest of souls. Christ-like power ministry in healing and miracles must punctuate the Gospel to bring the masses to Christ. This book seeks to help facilitate the Church's maturity in this matter and to hasten the coming of Christ for His prepared Bride, the Church.

Blessings!

Roger Sapp

---

[3] John 14:11-14

~1~

Christ Reveals the Father

The Foundation of Healing

There is a biblical truth that is a foundation to consistently healing the sick and injured. This foundational truth is frequently expressed in various ways in the New Testament. Many, who seem to generally accept the truth of divine healing, seem to fail in applying this foundational biblical truth to specific matters involving healing. Therefore, healing in any ministry that misses this truth is generally unpredictable, unreliable and inconsistent, if present at all. Failure to fully grasp this biblical truth hinders the efficient functioning of healing ministry and produces a weak theology that interferes with consistent faith for receiving and ministering healing.

The truth presented here is easily taken for granted because at first glance it seems so apparent and so biblically orthodox. Because it is so biblically orthodox, it can be easily underestimated in significance. Overlooking

7

and underestimating the significance of this truth continues to be the main reason why healing and miracle ministry is not found consistently in the lives of many Church leaders. Scanning to the last chapters of the book, without careful consideration of this foundational biblical truth, will cause the reader to understand only a portion of this essential matter.

There are many expressions of this foundational truth in Scripture. This chapter will present and review some of these.

Outlining This Foundational Truth

There are many places in the New Testament that express this important truth. However, the Gospel of John expresses it more often than any other book. Most of this chapter will center on the words of Christ in the Gospel of John, but will also review other parts of the New Testament, particularly the writings of the apostle Paul. Let's begin with a conversation between Christ and His disciple Philip found in the Gospel of John.

> *Jesus said to him, "I am the way, and the truth, and the life; no one comes to the Father, but through Me. If you had known Me, you would have known My Father also; from now on you know Him, and have seen Him." John 14:6-7*

These general truths emerge and will have application as the larger context of this passage is reviewed.

8

- *I am the way, the truth and the life; no one comes to the Father but through Me.*

Christ is the way, the truth and the life. While having a larger application than just healing ministry, Christ is also the way and the truth about healing. Christ's life produces healing. Any teaching on healing that does not find its basis in the life, ministry, death and resurrection of Christ will not be the truth. There is hardly a believer anywhere that would object to these rather obvious truths. However, the implications of these simple but profound words of Christ have yet to be considered.

- *If you had known Me, you would have known My Father also; from now on you know Him, and have seen Him.*

To know Christ is to know the Father. Studying the life of Christ will reveal the Father in matters of healing just as in all matters. If Christians fail to believe that Christ knows the Father's will and expresses it perfectly, healing will remain a puzzle that only occasionally gets solved.

In all matters, the Lord Jesus Christ ultimately reveals the will of the Father. While the entire Bible declares God's will and purpose, much of that purpose was unclear and unrevealed until Christ's example, teaching, and His sacrifice came on the scene of history. Mysteries that were once hidden are *now revealed in Christ*, particularly by Christ's example and words. The conversation between Philip and Christ continues with these thoughts:

9

Philip said to Him, "Lord, show us the Father, and it is enough for us." Jesus said to him, "Have I been so long with you, and yet you have not come to know Me, Philip? He who has seen Me has seen the Father; how do you say, 'Show us the Father'? Do you not believe that I am in the Father, and the Father is in Me? The words that I say to you I do not speak on My own initiative, but the Father abiding in Me does His works." John 14:8 10

This conversation reveals some important truths that will have application in the ministry of healing.

- _He who has seen Me has seen the Father._

Christ tells Philip that when He (Christ) is seen, the Father is seen. Every verbal expression of Christ and every action of Christ reveals the will of the Father.

- _I am in the Father and the Father is in Me._

The special nature of the relationship between Christ and the Father is the focus of this passage. Christ is in the Father and the Father is in Christ. Later in this passage, Christ says that believers must believe in this special relationship to do His works--including healing the sick and injured.

- *I don't speak on my own initiative.*

The Father abiding in Christ gives the words to Christ. The implication is that the teaching of Christ reveals the Father's perfect will in all matters including healing.

- *The Father abiding in Me does the works.*

Jesus gives credit to the Father for His works. The miracles and healing in the life of Christ were expressions of the divine purpose of the Father. Later in this passage, Christ reveals that it is essential to believe that the Father is doing His works in and through Christ if believers want to do the same kind of works.

Finally, in this conversation between Christ and Philip, Christ reveals what this special relationship between Him and His Father will mean to His disciples in the future. These are the most important verses in the exposition so far.

> *"Believe Me that I am in the Father, and the Father in Me; otherwise believe on account of the works themselves. Truly, truly, I say to you, he who believes in Me, the works that I do shall he do also; and greater works than these shall he do; because I go to the Father. And whatever you ask in My name, that will I do, that the Father may be glorified in the Son." John 14:11-13*

In these verses, Christ provides some important elements to entering a supernatural ministry like His own. He says:

- *Believe Me that I am in the Father…*

Faith in Christ includes believing that *He was and is in the Father*. This phrase is exceedingly important for consistent results in healing. In context of these verses, Christ has been teaching the importance of believing that He has been revealing the Father. In fact, Christ commands His followers to believe that very thing. If believers fail to believe that Christ reveals the will and the nature of the Father, they will find that faith will be difficult for many of the things that Christ did.

- *…Otherwise believe on the account of the works themselves…*

Understanding that Christ was expressing the fundamental will and purpose of the Father can be discerned by observing the works of Christ. Again, Christ encourages His followers to faith that He is expressing the will of the Father.

- *…he who believes in Me, the works that I do, He shall do also…*

This great promise is conditioned on the earlier statement that believers must believe that Christ is in the Father and the Father in Christ. If believers express the will of the Father as Christ did, they will do these same works.

This explains why believers must believe that Christ is expressing the will of the Father.

- *...and greater works than these shall he do; because I go to the Father...*

The promise of Christ that believers would do *greater works* is *conditioned* upon believing that Christ is in the Father and the Father is in Christ. Believers must believe that the will of the Father was finding absolute perfect expression in the actions, attitudes, teaching and commands of Jesus Christ. Now that Christ has gone to the Father, the same will of the Father is finding expression through believers empowered by the Spirit of Christ.

Believers can draw these important conclusions from this key passage:

> **Believing that God the Father was in Christ expressing His perfect will in teaching, attitudes, actions, and miraculous works is fundamental to accomplishing similar and even greater things in ministry. While many believers would give quick assent to this, if they fail to grasp the foundational significance of this essential matter, they will fail to experience the miraculous works that Christ promises.**

Much theology and practice today seems to fail to grasp this essential matter, and as a result, fails to *duplicate Christ's supernatural ministry*. Later in this book, the exposition will reveal that *duplication* is exactly what God desires as the Church enters the final harvest at the end of the age. Since this foundational matter is so important, we will review additional places in Scripture which discuss it.

Working the Works of God

A passage with some similar thoughts is found in Chapter 6 of John's Gospel. In this passage, Christ is asked an important question that relates to healing the sick:

> ... *"What shall we do, that we may work the works of God?" Jesus answered and said to them, "This is the work of God, that you believe in Him whom He has sent." John 6:28b-29*

The question could be rephrased to ask:

> ***What does it take to minister consistently like Christ in supernatural healing and miracle ministry?***

The answer is that believers must *believe in Him who He has sent.* The last part of the answer is more important than the first part. Believers are to *believe in Christ as the one that the Father has sent.* Again, the essential element is seeing the Father in Jesus Christ's actions, attitudes, words, works and commands. This is fundamental to *working the works of God. Believing* or *faith* is the essential element in each of the passages that have been considered. However, it is not a general unspecified *faith in Christ* but rather *faith that Christ is revealing the Father* that is significant.

Determining the Will of God the Father

Consider that Jesus Himself repeatedly stated that His actions demonstrated the will of the Father. For instance, Jesus said this about His actions and teaching in relationship with His Father.

> *"...I do nothing on My own initiative, but I speak these things as the Father taught Me. And He who sent Me is with Me; He has not left Me alone, for I always do the things that are pleasing to Him."* *John 8:28b-29*

From this short passage, these three important elements are revealed:

- *Actions.* Christ did not initiate the things that He did. This certainly includes healing and miracles. These events are expressions of the Father's will. Therefore, to learn about the Father's will in healing, believers need to carefully *observe the actions* of the Lord Jesus Christ as He dealt with sickness and disease.

- *Teaching.* Christ only spoke those things that the Father taught Him. This includes the teaching Christ did about healing. To learn about the Father's perfect will in healing, believers must study *what Christ said* about healing. Modern theology often ignores or reduces what Christ says about healing or what He says to people before and after they have been healed.

- *How to please the Father.* Christ only did things that pleased the Father. Therefore, the various healings and miracles, were pleasing to the Father. In order to *learn what pleases the Father* in matters of healing, believers need to study *the teaching of Christ and His actions* in these matters. Furthermore, believers need to recognize what Christ *did not say* and *did not do* in these matters. Teaching that advocates ideas, attitudes, and actions that do not find their basis in Christ Himself, will not please the Father. Therefore, comparison of modern teaching and attitudes about healing with Christ's teaching, attitudes and actions is highly appropriate and will be discussed throughout this book.

A Quick Look at Other Passages

Should these words of Christ be insufficient to convince the reader that Christ is the example and teacher in all matters and especially concerning healing and miracles, consider His words repeatedly on this matter.

> *Jesus therefore answered and was saying to them, "Truly, truly, I say to you, the Son can do nothing of Himself, unless it is something He sees the Father doing; for whatever the Father does, these things the Son also does in like manner. For the Father loves the Son, and shows Him all things that He Himself is doing; and greater works than these will He show Him, that you may marvel." John 5:19-20*

The ongoing, intimate relationship between Christ and the Father is apparent in this passage. However, some of the same truths that have been seen previously are also apparent.

- *...the Son can do nothing of Himself, unless it is something He sees the Father doing...*

Christ always revealed the Father's will in His actions, attitudes and teaching. Christ had revelation of what the Father wanted, and He lived out that revelation.

- *...for whatever the Father does, these things the Son also does in like manner.*

The truth of the ongoing intimacy between Christ and the Father is apparent in this passage. However, some have misunderstood this passage to think that if they do not *see* something that the Father is doing when a sick person is present that they cannot heal them. This is a serious misunderstanding of Christ's healing ministry. Christ had *previously seen* the Father healing the sick through Him. He had *already understood* the Father's will in healing the sick. He had a revelation of the Father's will in the matter. He understood this to be the *ongoing will* of the Father.

As Christ acted upon what He had *previously seen* the Father doing, He received *more specifics* from the Father on these matters for specific people. However, most people were healed in Christ's ministry in a relatively normal way without Him receiving a specific unusual revelation. Where a special revelation was received, the Gospel writers record it.

- *For the Father loves the Son, and shows Him all things that He Himself is doing...*

The intimacy of the relationship between the Father and the Son is revealed in many verses. Christ then demonstrated that He understood the Father's heart in His healing and delivering the afflicted around Him.

- ..._and greater works than these will He show Him, that you may marvel._

The _greater works_ of Christ were His expression of the heart of the Father towards people. Christ's revelation of the Father finds many other expressions in John's Gospel. For instance, Christ said:

> _"For I have come down from heaven, not to do My own will, but the will of Him (the Father) who sent Me." John 6:38_

In other words, should one wish to know the will of God the Father concerning a matter, his first observations should concern the life and words of Jesus Christ. Christ expressed this so often that it is amazing it is so often overlooked or seen as unimportant. For instance, He said:

> _"I can do nothing on My own initiative. As I hear, I judge; and My judgment is just, because I do not seek My own will, but the will of Him who sent Me." John 5:30_

And again, Christ said:

> _"but He who sent Me is true; and the things which I heard from Him,...I speak to the world." They did_

not realize that He had been speaking to them about the Father. John 8:26-27

Christ even described Himself to His enemies as a man who told the truth which was obtained from the Father:

> *"...a man who has told you the truth, which I heard from God..." John 8:40*

...and in a prayer to the Father, Christ stated that what He said was the Father's word:

> *"I have given them Thy word". John 17:14*

Christ repeatedly said that He knows the Father and was sent by the Father:

> *"I know Him; because I am from Him, and He sent Me." John 7:29*

Christ insisted on His intimacy with the Father:

> *"...even as the Father knows Me and I know the Father..." John 10:15a*

Christ's life was a ongoing expression of knowing the Father's heart and doing His word.

> *"...I know Him (the Father) and keep His (the Father's) Word..." John 8:55*

The works that Christ accomplished were the Father's will expressed openly.

> *"...for the works which the Father has given Me to accomplish, the very works that I do, bear witness of Me, that the Father has sent Me. And the Father who sent Me, He has borne witness of Me..."*
> *John 5:36b-37a*

The events that Christ accomplished were the work of the Father and His will being expressed:

> *"My food is to do the will of Him who sent Me and accomplish His work."* *John 4:34*

Few doubt the historical evidence that John's Gospel was the last book of the Bible written. It is significant that these last words of the New Testament written to the Church have so much emphasis on *believing* that *Christ was a pure reflection of the Father's will*. Believers who fail to grasp how significant this truth is, will never approach the consistency in the supernatural that Christ had while on earth. Christ repeatedly stated that this specific kind of believing is the key to *working the works of God*.

Other New Testament Expressions of This Truth

Other New Testament writers also expressed this important revealing relationship between God the Father and the Lord Jesus Christ. For instance, the apostle Paul tells us about this relationship in Colossians.

Christ Reveals the Father's Will

And He (Christ) is the image of the invisible God...
Colossians 1:15

This simple phrase means that when believers see Christ in the New Testament, they are seeing what God, the Father is like. A similar truth is found in the same letter a few verses later. There Paul says:

For in Him (Christ) all the fullness of Deity dwells in bodily form... Colossians 2:9

A concise explanation of this verse is simply that God the Father was present in Christ as He demonstrated the Father's will in words, attitudes, actions and works. Christ was an ongoing revelation of the Father in every way possible.

The writer of the Book of Hebrews also introduces his book with a similar message about Christ's revelation of the Father.

God, after He spoke long ago to the fathers in the prophets in many portions and in many ways, in these last days has spoken to us in His Son, whom He (the Father) appointed heir of all things, through whom also He (the Father) made the world. And He (Jesus Christ) is the radiance of His (the Father's) glory and the exact representation of His (the Father's) nature... Hebrews 1:1-3a[1]

---

[1]Words in parenthesis added by author for emphasis and clarity

This passage reveals Christ's preeminence in powerful ways:

- *...in these last days has spoken to us in His Son...*

The author of Hebrews offers a powerful comparison in these words. He reminds us that God spoke previously through the Old Testament prophets in various ways. However, something greater, something more substantial has happened now. The author of Hebrews states that having the Son of God speak now is a higher and more complete revelation of the Father. The next few phrases in this passage tell us of Christ's involvement in the creation of the world and indicates the superiority of Christ's revelation to the previous Old Testament prophets speaking. Then the author of Hebrews reveals more about Christ.

- *...and He (Jesus Christ) is the radiance of His (the Father's) glory...*

Radiance is a good translation of what the Greek manuscripts say here. Other possible translations would say that Christ is the *shining forth* or *reflection* of the *glory* of the Father. The truth that the careful examination of Christ's life results in discovery of the Father again emerges in Hebrews. What a powerful pronouncement of the superiority of Christ's revelation!

- *...and the exact representation of His (the Father's) nature...*

Here the Greek word translated *exact representation* is somewhat familiar to English speakers. It is the Greek word *charakter*. This is source of the English word *character*. The Greek word finds its origin in the making of coins by striking them, thus creating an impression upon them. This word can be translated as *coined impression* or *exact reproduction* of the Father's nature. The Greek word translated *nature* can be translated as *real substance* or *essence*. In other words, what these opening verses in Hebrews are telling us is that Christ is the exact representation, the coined impression, and the exact reproduction of the nature, real substance, and essence of the Father. No one ever revealed the Father perfectly in every way until Christ. Therefore, no theology of healing should ever be formed without careful consideration of Christ's healing ministry.

A Christocentric Theology of Healing

Healing was demonstrated throughout the Old Testament. However, a clear theology cannot be founded upon these examples. Healing is also revealed in the lives of the apostles, in the Book of Acts and mentioned in various places in the Letters of Paul and others. However, a theology of healing cannot be properly formed from these alone. The foundation of a proper theology of healing must be built on Christ alone. Only then can a structure of doctrine and practice be built properly.

The Old Testament and the Letters of various apostles and other First Century Christian leaders cannot be properly interpreted without clear understanding of what Jesus taught and demonstrated in the matter of healing. This is generally called in theological terms as *C*hristocentric theology. This simply means that theology is centered upon and founded upon Christ Himself. Any theology that does not find this kind of relationship with Christ should not really be considered *Christian.* Unfortunately, there is much theology involving healing that seems to ignore the example and teaching of Christ Himself. Therefore, much theology of healing is not entirely *Christocentric,* and therefore does not clearly express the will of God. Because these murky theologies do not clearly express the will of the Father in these matters, and they encourage attitudes that do not emulate Christ, those that embrace them are relatively powerless to help people in the same ways that Christ helped people.

Surely, no Christian would attempt to form a theology of salvation without Christ Himself being the primary consideration in that theology. However, there seem to be serious attempts to form theologies of healing without Christ being central. Forming a theology of healing without making Christ the foundation is like trying to form a Christian theology of salvation from the Law of Moses. While the Law of Moses *is* God's Word, the Law cannot be understood or taught properly without the cross of Christ being a first consideration. Forming a theology of healing without Christ is similar to attempting to form a theology of salvation without the sacrifice of Christ at Calvary.

Some sincere leaders who have rejected theological positions that they once held such as Dispensationalism or

Cessationism[2], still seem to retain much of the reasoning and attitudes that seem to accompany those false doctrines. This reasoning and attitudes effectively robs them of faith for healing. Some of these leaders seem to have a *cessationist hangover* that affects their theology specifically in the matter of healing and miracles. Yet God's Word clearly states,

> *Jesus Christ is the same yesterday and today, yes and forever. Hebrews 13:8*

Christ is ignored or minimized in the formation of their theology of healing. Some see Christ as a *special case* and not as revealing the will of the Father in these matters for us today. Some seem to be able to ignore the words of Christ about healing and miracles. All this produces some bad theology that focuses on Job's suffering and Paul's thorn in the flesh. Sadly, when someone is seriously ill, often a message of suffering and death is presented rather than a message about the life, the healing and delivering power of Christ.

This less than Christocentric theology leaves us with an unsolvable puzzle about God's will in healing. In turn, this murky theology creates an ineffective ministry to

---

[2] Dispensationalism and Cessationism both teach that God is no longer working the same ways that He worked in the New Testament. In other words, these theological positions teach that the New Testament is a reflection of how God has worked in the past and not how He is presently working. These theological positions, while stating that the New Testament is inspired, teach that most of the supernatural aspects of the New Testament such as healing and miracle ministry is not for today. See the author's book **The Last Apostles on Earth** for more information on these erroneous but popular theological positions.

others in need of healing by creation of an atmosphere of doubt. This atmosphere of doubt is reinforced by examples and reasoning about why God does not heal. It suggests that suffering, pain, disability and untimely death might somehow be better and a mysterious blessing from God.

The consideration in the next chapters will be narrowly focusing upon what Scripture reveals concerning healing. Therefore, it is entirely appropriate to examine healing in the ministry of Christ. As the chapters of this book unfold, the reader will consider every pertinent verse dealing directly with healing in the New Testament and some in the Old Testament. However, the book will first consider the examples and teaching of Christ contained in the Gospel accounts to instruct us as to the will of God the Father. General descriptions of the ministry of Christ to the multitudes will be considered first. Then, descriptions of Christ's ministry to specific individuals will be considered. Where it is appropriate to build upon the foundation of Christ, the ministries of Christ's disciples will be reviewed also.

Section 1

General Descriptions of Christ's & His Disciples' Healing & Miracle Ministry to the Multitudes

~2~

Christ's Ministry to the Masses in Matthew and Mark

As discussed in Chapter One, the New Testament teaches that Christ reveals the Father. Observation of Christ's works, actions, attitudes and teaching concerning healing reveals the will of the Father in these matters. The will of the Father ought to be clear to believers since there is an abundant amount of scriptural information about healing in the ministry of Christ. If people were *clean-slates* unaffected by any view other than Scripture, this would be true. However, most readers in the United States, even those who are not familiar with the New Testament, come to this subject with predetermined views that often prevent or limit healing ministry. Often they are reacting to extreme positions and reject the truth because it may have some similarities to an apparent extreme. One of the objectives of this book is to analyze the New Testament passages that relate to healing so we may determine what actually is and is not there. It is important to discover what culture, religious tradition and unbelieving theologies have overlooked, imposed or dismissed from the New Testament accounts of Christ's healing ministry.

This study begins with those accounts in the Gospels of Matthew and Mark which are *general descriptions* of the healing and miracle ministry of Christ. *A general description is a passage where Christ is dealing with a group of people rather than an individual. In other* words, these are descriptions of Christ's ministry to the *masses*. The specific events and individuals that were healed will be considered in later chapters.

General Descriptions in Matthew's Gospel

General descriptions that contain a great deal of information about Christ's healing ministry are found in all three Synoptic Gospels and in a lessor degree in John's Gospel and the Book of Acts. Christ fully expresses the will of the Father in these passages, which we will review in the order in which they appear in the New Testament. The first is found in Matthew's Gospel, Chapter 4.

> *And Jesus was going about in all Galilee, teaching in their synagogues, and proclaiming the Gospel of the kingdom, and healing every kind of disease and every kind of sickness among the people. And the news about Him went out into all Syria; and they brought to Him all who were ill, taken with various diseases and pains, demoniacs, epileptics, paralytics; and He healed them. Matthew 4:23-24*

Christ's Ministry to the Masses
in Matthew and Mark

There is a great amount of important information in these two verses.

- *And Jesus was going about in all Galilee, teaching in their synagogues, and proclaiming the Gospel of the kingdom...*

The activity of healing in the ministry of Christ is found often in a context of traveling, teaching and proclaiming the Gospel of the kingdom of God. The word *proclaiming* is translated *preaching* in some versions. Later in this book, the subject of proclaiming or preaching the Gospel will be considered in detail.

- *...and healing every kind of disease and every kind of sickness among the people.*

Matthew, one of the twelve original apostles and an eyewitness of the ministry of Christ, reveals that Christ healed *every kind of disease and sickness*. No disease or sickness was excluded. This is significant information in determining the will of the Father in healing. What is absent or missing in these accounts is significant as well. No one appears to be excluded because of judgment, a mysterious discipline of God, a mysterious blessing from God or any other reason. Christ does not separate the ill and injured people into categories of those who should be healed and those who should not be healed.

- *...and they brought to Him all who were ill, taken with various diseases and pains, demoniacs, epileptics, paralytics; and He healed them.*

The description of the kinds of problems and people that Christ healed seems to expand to cover *five* various types of problems: disease, pains, demoniacs, epileptics and paralytics. It is interesting that those who were in pain were a special category of those Christ healed. The passage also strongly implies that *all* that were *brought to Him* were *healed.*

- *Absent from the account.* What is absent in this general account is any *hesitation* in the ministry of Christ toward healing the sick. There is no evaluation of the will of God in each situation for each person. Christ *already knows* what the Father wants. The Father wants to heal. There seems to be no separation of people into categories of those who should be healed and those who should not be healed.

Matthew's Second General Description

The second general description of the ministry of Christ to the masses is found in Chapter 9 of Matthew's Gospel. It contains an important quotation from the Old Testament Book of Isaiah.

> *And when evening had come, they brought to Him many who were demon-possessed; and He cast out the spirits with a word, and healed all who were ill in order that what was spoken through Isaiah the prophet might be fulfilled, saying, "HE HIMSELF*

TOOK OUR INFIRMITIES, AND CARRIED AWAY OUR DISEASES." Matthew 8:16-17

These things are notable in this passage:

- *...they brought to Him many who were demon-possessed; and He cast out the spirits with a word...*

Christ cast out demons through a *word* implies that He was verbally commanding them to leave. This method of casting out demons also appears later in the ministry of the twelve apostles, Paul and others in Scripture. While there are other means of deliverance, this is the ordinary way to cast out demons today.

- *...and healed all who were ill...*

This is very clear. All were healed that had been brought to Him. There was no division of people into those who should be healed by Christ and those who should not be healed. Considering that there were *many* brought to Him, there is no evidence that even a few of them were being helped by their sickness or that their sickness was doing a mysterious good work in them. Since Christ healed *all* that were ill among the *many*, it must have been the Father's will for them all to be well. Not a single person among the *many* here was demonstrating sickness as the will of the Father.

- *...in order that what was spoken through Isaiah the prophet might be fulfilled...*

31

Performing Miracles and Healing

Matthew reveals that this example of healing ministry fulfilled the prophecy found in the Book of Isaiah, Chapter 53. This prophecy is highly significant because it predicts the redemptive, atoning work of the Savior at the cross hundreds of years before Christ's birth.

- _...(the prophet Isaiah) saying, "HE HIMSELF TOOK OUR INFIRMITIES, AND CARRIED AWAY OUR DISEASES."_

These words from the Book of Isaiah 53:4 are quoted by the apostle Matthew. The context of the entire passage of Isaiah Chapter 53 describes the sacrificial work of Jesus Christ. In other words, this passage substantiates that when Christ died for our sins at the cross, He also _died for our infirmities and diseases_. Fully embracing the truth that healing is in the atoning work of the cross is also significant in producing consistent results in healing ministry.

- _Absent from the account_: Notably absent is the teaching and preaching of the Gospel of the kingdom. Often, these three elements are together: the message of the kingdom, healing and casting out demons. Nonetheless, it is possible to heal the sick or cast out demons without the proclamation of the kingdom. Also absent from this account is anyone not being healed. From anyone's way of accounting, the Father's will was to heal all that came to Christ in this particular situation.

Christ's Ministry to the Masses in Matthew and Mark

Matthew's Third General Description

The third general description of the healing ministry of Christ to the masses in Matthew's Gospel is not quite as detailed. However, this account does reinforce a few of the same facts:

> *And Jesus was going about all the cities and the villages, teaching in their synagogues, and proclaiming the Gospel of the kingdom, and healing every kind of disease and every kind of sickness. Matthew 9:35*

Some of the same biblical facts are discovered here:

- *...proclaiming the Gospel of the kingdom...*

Healing in this situation occurred in the context of public proclamation and teaching the kingdom of God.

- *...healing every kind of disease and every kind of sickness...*

Christ healed every kind of disease and every kind of sickness. This logically implies that all were healed since no sickness or disease was left out. There did not seem to be the same sort of limitations, concerns, fears of excess and fears of failure displayed in Christ's ministry that seems to be imposed by some modern theologies upon those who seek to heal the sick today. Clearly, an identical ministry to Christ's would be rejected and criticized in many Churches today. Some Christian ministers today react strongly against any ministry similar to Christ's ministry to the afflicted. These ministers consider this kind of ministry dangerous and excessive. These ministers have adjusted themselves to powerlessness. However, because the end of the age is drawing near, things are changing dramatically. The supernatural ministry of Christ is being _duplicated_ and experienced in many places as it should. Nothing less will produce the great harvest at the end of the age.

Matthew's Fourth General Description

The fourth general description of the healing ministry of Christ is found in Matthew's Gospel, Chapter 15. These events happened along the Sea of Galilee just before the miracle of the feeding of the four thousand. In fact, the people who were healed in these verses were included in the miracle of the four thousand.

> _And great multitudes came to Him, bringing with them those who were lame, crippled, blind, dumb, and many others, and they laid them down at His feet; and He healed them, so that the multitude marveled as they saw the dumb speaking, the crippled restored, and the lame walking, and the blind seeing; and they glorified the God of Israel._ _Matthew 15:30-31_

This passage has some important truth to discern.

- _And great multitudes came to Him, bringing with them those who were lame, crippled, blind, dumb, and many others, and they laid them down at His feet..._

The next verses beyond this passage describe the miracle of the feeding of the four thousand. That passage reveals that there were *four thousand men, besides women and children*[1] present. Since the women were not being counted in the four thousand, this means that there were a least six thousand adults present, probably more. In any case, this large group of people could have brought hundreds of adults and children with them who needed healing. If the estimate is correct, some simple math can be done. If only *one out of ten* healthy adults brought someone needing healing, then there were more than *six hundred people with healing needs* in this one situation. This should be a conservative estimation. There were probably many more.

This passage does not focus so much on sickness as it does on disabling conditions. Four kinds of disabled people were brought to Jesus that are named: *The lame, the crippled, the blind and the dumb*. In English, it may be difficult to distinguish between the *lame* and the *crippled*. Generally speaking, the New American Standard does a wonderful job in expressing the actual Greek. It is perhaps the most reliable of all modern English version available. However, in this case, the word *crippled* would be better translated as *maimed or injured* to avoid confusion with the word *lame*.

The grammar of this passage indicates that there was more than one of each of the four specific kinds

---

[1] Matthew 15:38

disabled people. The passage also allows for all other kinds of sickness and disease being healed in this group by using the phrase *and many others*. This adds a fifth category that includes all kinds of sickness.

Using simple math again and the previous estimate of 600 people, this group can be divided by the five categories and determine that *on average* that there was more than a hundred of each of the five kinds of conditions. Of course, this is modest speculation based on assumptions on the facts revealed in this passage. There is no way to actually know the real numbers but there is reasonable and logical evidence of a great number of people being healed here from the information given in the passage.

- *...and He healed them, so that the multitude marveled as they saw the dumb speaking, the crippled restored, and the lame walking, and the blind seeing; and they glorified the God of Israel.*

Christ healed this large group of disabled and sick people in the presence of thousands of other people. Potentially hundreds of sick, injured and disabled people were healed in this situation. Christ wanted to feed the more than four thousand people there because they had been when Him for more than three days indicates that the healing ministry to so many took a long time to finish.

This passage does not reveal anyone not being healed or being sent away for any reason. Surely there would have been *at least a few* in the mix of hundreds of sick, injured and disabled people that Christ would have allowed to remain in that condition *if* that condition was actually the Father's will for them. However, this passage and many others, will show that the Father's will for the sick, injured and disabled is wholeness. Christ demonstrates the will of the Father in this matter of healing repeatedly.

Mark's General Descriptions

The fifth general description of the healing ministry of Jesus Christ to the masses is found in Mark, Chapter 1.

> *And when evening had come, after the sun had set, they began bringing to Him all who were ill and those who were demon-possessed. And the whole city had gathered at the door. And He healed many who were ill with various diseases, and cast out many demons; and He was not permitting the demons to speak, because they knew who He was. Mark 1:32-34*

This passage has more emphasis on casting out demons than has been seen in the passages in Matthew's Gospel.

- *...they began bringing to Him all who were ill and those who were demon-possessed.*

This is a similar description as previous passages. The ill and demonized were brought to Christ. This implies that many were too ill or demonized to come on their own. Healing and casting out demons are again found together.

- _...And He healed many who were ill with various diseases..._

Christ healed _many_ in this passage. The passage _does not say_ that _all_ were healed. On the other hand, it _does not say_ that some were _not healed_ either. It is impossible to tell by the statement here if all were healed. However, there is _not a hint_ of separation of the sick people into classes of those who should be healed and those who should not be healed. Unfortunately, popular modern theology suggests that the Father's will does separate people into classes in matters of healing.

Unbelieving theology wants to find _many not being healed_ in Mark's description. However, what the passage actual says is that _many were healed_. It says nothing about anyone not being healed. It is unlikely that Mark was trying to indicate anything about anyone not being healed. Even if Mark was trying to indicate that some were not healed, then logically the opposite of _many being healed_ is a _few not being healed_. If allowance is made for the possibility that a _few were not healed_, this does not indicate that the Father's will for the _few_ was sickness. The Father's will is _not fulfilled_ in _many important matters_ for various reasons. If the Father's will were always fulfilled, then everyone in the world would be saved and certainly delivered from demons. If the Father's will were always fulfilled, then no one would die because of some drunk driver. If the Father's will were always fulfilled, then no child would suffer physical or sexual abuse or go to bed hungry. Therefore, someone not being healed on any particular occasion *does not reveal* that remaining in that condition is the Father's will for that person. There is certainly nothing in this passage to support the idea that it might have been the will of the Father not to heal some.

- *...and cast out many demons; and He was not permitting the demons to speak, because they knew who He was...*

This passage reveals more about casting out demons than the two previous passages. Obviously, the demons wanted to speak but Christ was not permitting them to do so. The two ministries, healing and casting out demons, were common elements in the ministry of Christ and His followers. These two elements of ministry are also common in the ministry of the twelve apostles, Paul and others and should be common elements of ministry today.

Sickness, injury and demonic activity are *always* treated as *enemies* of humanity everywhere in the four Gospels. Friendship with sickness and disease are not found in the New Testament. Nothing that Christ says would encourage believers to have any other approach than seeking to heal and deliver the sick, injured and demonized. Other approaches come from misguided theology and the unbelieving traditions of men.

Mark's Second General Description
Another passage in Mark's Gospel has some general statements about Christ's ministry. It is found in Chapter 3

and is the sixth general description of the healing ministry of Christ to the masses:

> *And He told His disciples that a boat should stand ready for Him because of the multitude, in order that they might not crowd Him; for He had healed many, with the result that all those who had afflictions pressed about Him in order to touch Him. And whenever the unclean spirits beheld Him, they would fall down before Him and cry out, saying, "You are the Son of God!" Mark 3:9-11*

There are several things extremely worthy of additional comment in this passage:

- *...a boat should stand ready for Him because of the multitude, in order that they might not crowd Him; for He had healed many...*

So many people were being healed that a multitude seeking healing began to crowd Christ. The passage again uses the term *many,* which does not reveal if *all* were being healed. However, this passage does not imply that some were not healed either. There is simply no way to know with certainty from the words here. In fact, when compared with the information in other passages concerning healing, it is extremely doubtful that Mark was trying to reveal to his readers that some were not healed. However, later in this chapter a passage will be reviewed in Mark where some were not healed who perhaps should have been.

Christ's Ministry to the Masses
in Matthew and Mark

- *...for He had healed many, with the result that all those who had afflictions pressed about Him in order to touch Him...*

The *laying on of hands* was a common way that Christ healed this sick. However, this passage reveals another common way that healing was administered in Christ's ministry. These people were being healed *from touching Christ* rather than Him touching them. This is revealed in a number of other passages as well. Later in this study, specific people described by the Gospels in detail as being healed *by touching Christ* will be reviewed.

- *...And whenever the unclean spirits beheld Him, they would fall down before Him and cry out, saying, "You are the Son of God!"*

In an earlier passage, Christ was not allowing the demons to speak. Perhaps this was the reason; He didn't want demons to proclaim His deity.

General Description of Some Not Healed

Mark's Gospel does record a general description of Christ's ministry to the masses where there were evidently people who were sick that were not healed. The context of this passage is in his hometown and where people have reacted to Him in unbelief. In this circumstance, Christ announced that He was *a prophet without honor*. This passage is found in Mark Chapter 6 and is the seventh general description of the healing ministry of Christ to the masses.

> _...many listeners were astonished, saying, "Where did this man get these things, and what is this wisdom given to Him, and such miracles as these performed by His hands? Is not this the carpenter, the son of Mary...?" And they took offense at Him...and He could do no miracle there except that He laid His hands upon a few sick people and healed them. And He wondered at their unbelief..._
> _Mark 6:2b-6a_

This passage has some unique points to draw from the ministry of Christ to the masses that have not been considered:

- _...And they took offense at Him._

Even the perfect and compassionate Son of God was unable to please everyone. Even those in His own hometown and among His family did not understand Him or His mission and therefore were offended. They were offended because someone they thought they knew well was doing miracles. They were focused on His humanity and did not see that He was revealing the will and power of the Father. Unfortunately, the great blessing of healing ministry often comes with misunderstanding and offense even for the most sensitive of Christ's servants. Rejection and misunderstanding from a few people is a small price to pay for the capacity to help many suffering people.

- _And He could do no miracle there except that He laid His hands upon a few sick people and healed them._

Christ's Ministry to the Masses
in Matthew and Mark

Christ was much less able, comparatively powerless, to help people in His own hometown. There is no mention of the people of His hometown coming to Him. In fact, the context reveals that their very familiarity with Him created unbelief and offense in them. The statement in this passage also reveals that the normal and routine ministry of Christ was to be able to perform miracles and healing.

- *And He wondered at their unbelief...*

What was different in this circumstance that created the seemingly powerlessness of Christ to help these people? It was simply their surprising *unbelief.* Those that believed that Christ could help them flocked to Him in multitudes. Conversely, the reaction of the people in Christ's hometown was basically... *What's the big deal? We know all about this guy.* Because of their lack of faith, He was only able to help a few sick people and was unable to do any miracles. This event is entirely consistent with Christ's verbal teaching on healing which will be observed in subsequent chapters.

~3~

Christ's Ministry to the Masses in Luke, John & Acts

General Accounts in the Gospel of Luke

By far, the Gospel of Luke contains more of the general descriptions of the healing ministry of Christ to the masses than the other Gospels. The first of these accounts is found in Luke Chapter 4. This is also the eighth general account found in the Gospels.

> *And while the sun was setting, all who had any sick with various diseases brought them to Him; and laying His hands on every one of them, He was healing them. Luke 4:40*

There are several important and familiar elements in these verses:

Performing Miracles and Healing

- _...all who had any sick with various diseases brought them to Him..._

The _all_ here apparently describes people who had family members and possibly friends who were sick. These relatives brought the sick to Christ.

- _...and laying His hands on every one of them, He was healing them._

Laying on hands was a very normal way for Christ to heal the sick, although it was not the only way. This statement also strongly implies that _every one_ was being healed that Christ laid His hands upon.

- _Absent from the account:_ As in the previous accounts, there is no revelation that the Father was doing anything mysterious or good in the lives of these people in the matter of sickness. When they encountered Christ, the Father revealed His will for them in healing. Christ never sends someone away with a deep theological explanation of how sickness was doing him or her some sort of good. Also absent is the proclamation of the Gospel. This book already noted that the proclamation of the Gospel does not always accompany healing in Christ's ministry. Christ repeatedly heals the sick and injured wherever and whenever they respond in faith to Him no matter what the circumstance.

Christ's Ministry to the Masses
in Luke, John and Acts

Luke's Second General Account

In the next chapter of Luke's Gospel, we find a general description of the ministry of Jesus Christ to the masses is found. It is also the ninth general account found in the Gospels.

> *But the news about Him was spreading even farther, and great multitudes were gathering to hear Him and to be healed of their sicknesses. But He Himself would often slip away to the wilderness and pray. Luke 5:15-16*

There are several things to observe in this passage:

- *...But the news about Him was spreading even farther, and great multitudes were gathering...*

This is similar to some of the previous passages that this book has reviewed. Christ was able to draw a *whole city*, a *multitude* in previous passages. Because healing needs are universal, any dynamic healing ministry will have the capacity to draw a crowd when people really believe something is genuinely happening. Therefore, healing ministry always has an evangelistic capacity that many other ministries lack.

- *...gathering to hear Him and to be healed of their sicknesses...*

This is a similar idea expressed in a different way. In earlier passages, Christ was teaching and proclaiming

47

the Gospel of the Kingdom of God. Luke observes that people were *gathering to hear Him*. Again, in combination with the Gospel of the Kingdom, He was healing the sick.

- *...But He Himself would often slip away to the wilderness and pray...*

This is an important ingredient in the ongoing power of Christ to help people. In order to have a ministry of power in public, Christ had a secret life of communion in prayer with the Father.

- *Absent from this passage:* There is no mention of a discerning of the will of the Father for separate people, or hesitation on the part of Jesus in healing anyone or anyone not being healed for any reason.

Luke's Third General Account

A third passage in Luke's Gospel is found in Chapter 6. It is also the tenth general description of the healing ministry of Christ to the masses found in the four Gospels. It is found a few verses after Luke reveals that *He (Christ) spent a night in prayer to God...*and then Christ selected His twelve disciples and took them with Him as He healed people:

> *And He descended with them (the twelve disciples), and stood on a level place; and there was a great multitude of His disciples, and a great throng of people from all Judea and Jerusalem and the coastal region of Tyre and Sidon, who had come to hear Him, and to be healed of their diseases; and*

those who were troubled with unclean spirits were being cured. And all the multitude were trying to touch Him, for power was coming from Him and healing them all. Luke 6:17-19

Consider these familiar truths and these new truths as the nature of Christ's healing ministry continues to be revealed in the Gospel of Luke.

- *...a great multitude of His disciples, and a great throng of people...*

The passage draws a distinction between the commitment level of the people coming to Jesus. Here, they are divided *into His disciples* and other *people.*

- *...who had come to hear Him, and to be healed of their diseases...*

While the passage draws a distinction between two groups of people, both groups have the same motive in coming to Christ. They wanted to *hear Him* and to *be healed.* This is familiar. The Gospel writers repeatedly report that healing and hearing the Gospel of the Kingdom of God were found together. Coming to *hear* and *be healed* are revealed here as a proper motives to come to Christ since the sick and afflicted received what they came for.

- *...and those who were troubled with unclean spirits were being cured.*

Luke, like Matthew and Mark, reveals that Christ's public ministry included casting out demons. In fact, preaching and teaching the Gospel of the Kingdom of God, healing the sick and casting out demons are the three ongoing, normal and expected expressions of Christ's ministry. Luke describes Christ's dealing with demons here as *curing* those who *were troubled with unclean spirits*. This reveals that some sickness, but not all, is caused by demons. This truth is also revealed in a number of specific events that we will review in future chapters.

- *And all the multitude were trying to touch Him, for power was coming from Him and healing them all.*

This situation was wonderfully dynamic. The people's faith in Christ as Healer was releasing great power to heal. Christ did not need to touch them. Instead they were touching Him and receiving from God. No person who came to touch Him was denied healing. It was the will of God for all to be healed in a multitude. This again reveals that the Father was not drawing distinctions between people seeking healing. All who believed could receive.

Luke's Fourth General Description

This eighth general description in the Gospels is interesting because it contains Christ's own description of His ministry.

And the disciples of John reported to him about all these things. And summoning two of his disciples, John sent them to the Lord, saying, "Are You the Expected One, or do we look for someone else?" And when the men had come to Him, they said, "John the Baptist has sent us to You, saying, 'Are You the Expected One, or do we look for someone else'?" At that very time He cured many people of diseases and afflictions and evil spirits; and He granted sight to many who were blind. And He answered and said to them, "Go and report to John what you have seen and heard: the BLIND RECEIVE SIGHT, the lame walk, the lepers are cleansed, and the deaf hear, the dead are raised up, the POOR HAVE THE GOSPEL PREACHED TO THEM. And blessed is he who keeps from stumbling over Me." Luke 7:18-23

The disciples of John the Baptist came to Christ with a significant question. Christ's response contains information on the kinds of attitudes that the Church should have toward healing and miracle ministry.

- *And when the men had come to Him, they said, "John the Baptist has sent us to You, saying, 'Are You the Expected One, or do we look for someone else?'"*

The context of this question reveals that the disciples of John the Baptist had observed the miracle ministry of Christ. John's disciples had reported to John what they had seen. In turn, John had sent a delegation back to Christ to ask Him if He was the *Expected One*. John was obviously referring to the much-prophesied coming of the Messiah (Christ). The delegation of John's disciples got another strong dose of miracles and healing in Christ's ministry as an answer.

- *At that very time He cured many people of diseases and afflictions and evil spirits; and He granted sight to many who were blind.*

51

Christ cured *many* of four kinds of conditions mentioned in this verse; diseases, afflictions, evil spirits and blindness. It particularly focuses on the *many* blind that were *granted sight* by Christ. This implies that He had some *control over healing* of the blindness and was able to *give sight* to the blind. Christ did not have total control since other passages reveal that He could not perform miracles under conditions of unbelief. However, since these people had exercised faith by coming to Christ for healing, they were all healed. This element of partial control is found in many other passages and is a key to understanding how healing works in practical ministry. This idea of partial control of healing is very contrary to most people's conceptions and therefore creates objections. Therefore, this whole realm deserves further exploration and explanation later in this book.

In the next portion of this passage, Christ tells John's disciples that what they have observed in His ministry is their answer. They should be able to identify that Jesus is the Messiah[1] by virtue of five kinds miraculous works and His preaching of the Gospel to the poor.

- ... *"Go and report to John what you have seen and heard: the BLIND RECEIVE SIGHT, the lame walk, the lepers are cleansed, and the deaf hear, the dead are raised up, the POOR HAVE THE GOSPEL PREACHED TO THEM.*

When the verses above are considered together, eight conditions are mentioned as being dealt with in Christ's

---

[1] Messiah and Christ are two transliterated words that come from Hebrew and Greek respectively. They both mean "the anointed one". For a more detailed explanation, see the author's book *The Last Apostles on Earth*, pages 51-62.

ministry. These conditions are *diseases, afflictions, evil spirits, blindness, lameness, leprosy, deafness, and death.* If Christ Himself places an emphasis on this aspect of His ministry, who today has authority to reduce this emphasis? Perhaps today, many lost persons do not really recognize Christ in His Church simply because the Church fails to represent Him properly. Believers fail to represent Christ by failing to demonstrate His miraculous works that would enable people to easily identify Him at work in His Church. Believers fail often because they are waiting for the Father to reveal His *already revealed* will. Believers fail to act in faith because of unmerited fears and unscriptural cautions about being presumptuous. Some cautions have the appearance of wisdom but do not stand up to examination when the supernatural ministry of Christ is used as the standard. The Holy Spirit is preparing a company of believers who will risk reputation and rejection of the religious establishment to do the Father's will. They will fearlessly minister like the Savior in the last days of this age. They will abandon all desire for honor from anyone besides God.

Luke's Fifth Description

Another general passage is found in Chapter 9. This twelfth general description found in the Gospels has familiar elements.

And taking them with Him, He privately withdrew to a city called Bethsaida. But the multitudes were aware of this and followed Him; and welcoming them, He began speaking to them about the

Performing Miracles and Healing

Kingdom of God and curing those who had need of healing. Luke 9:10b-11

This passage gives us some interesting insight into Christ's ongoing knowledge of how His ministry was to function.

- *He privately withdrew to a city called Bethsaida*

Sometimes Christ allowed the circumstances to dictate His ministry. In a time when Christ tried to quietly withdraw, He did not succeed. A group of people found Him.

- *But the multitudes were aware of this and followed Him...*

Christ gladly ministered to these people despite His plan to withdraw. For those who think that Christ must have had specific revelation for every moment of His ministry, this passage shows that He did not have prior knowledge or a specific revelation of the Father's will for these people but ministered to the sick as He had opportunity. Christ knew what the Father wanted for all the sick and injured. The Father wanted them well.

Christ had tried to privately withdraw to Bethsaida. Perhaps, He and His disciples needed a time of rest. However, the multitudes knew that He had gone to Bethsaida and sought out Christ. Repeatedly, as revealed in previous passages, there was always a time of healing when crowds of people sought out Christ.

- *...speaking to them about the kingdom of God...*

Again, healing is revealed in the context of preaching the Gospel of the Kingdom of God. While healing is sometimes found in these general passages without any reference to the Gospel of the Kingdom, it is frequently discovered where the Gospel of the Kingdom of God is being preached and taught.

- *...and curing those who had need of healing.*

This statement does not allow for some not being healed in this situation. Again, there is no separation of people into categories. Christ does not separate those who should be healed from those who should not be healed. The will of the Father being revealed by Christ is that the Father wants people well.

Luke's Sixth and Seventh Description

Luke's sixth general description is easily overlooked. In this verse, Luke describes the healing and miracles in Christ's ministry as *glorious things being done by Him.* Christ's healing of the afflicted and suffering is indeed glorious. This constitutes the thirteenth general description of Christ's healing ministry to the masses.

> *And as He said this, all His opponents were being humiliated; and the entire multitude was rejoicing over all the glorious things being done by Him. Luke 13:17*

A few verses later, Christ describes His ministry in unmistakable terms. In a reference that is the fourteenth general description, Christ tells someone to describe His ministry in a particular way to King Herod. Herod is described by Christ as *that fox*, which reveals that Christ was aware of Herod's political cunning, craftiness and ruthlessness.

> *And He said to them, "Go and tell that fox, 'Behold, I cast out demons and perform cures today and tomorrow, and the third day I reach My goal'."* Luke 13:32

In this verse, Christ describes His ministry in three parts; t*oday, tomorrow and the third da*y. The first and second days, Christ reveals that He *casts out demons and performs cures*. The third day is most likely a reference to the His death and resurrection. Christ says that on the *third day He reaches His goal*. It appears here that Christ felt *casting out demons* and *performing cures* were representative of two-thirds of His ministry. The idea of *performing cures* is also important. This idea of *performing* will be discussed in detail in the general descriptions of Christ's healing ministry to the masses found in John's Gospel.

Before moving to the general descriptions found in John's Gospel, an organizational comment needs to be made here. Luke is the author of two books of the New Testament and both contain general descriptions of Christ's ministry. Two general descriptions of Christ's ministry are found in the Book of Acts. These two descriptions of the supernatural ministry of Christ to the masses will be considered at the end of this chapter. They are placed at the end of this chapter to maintain the order in which they appear in the New Testament.

General Descriptions in John's Gospel

John's Gospel has a few verses that are general descriptions of the healing and miracle ministry of Jesus Christ. Unfortunately, they are not as detailed and, therefore, are less helpful overall. The first of these is found in Chapter 6 and is the fifteenth general description to the masses found in the Gospels.

> *And a great multitude was following Him, because they were seeing the signs which He was performing on those who were sick. John 6:2*

There are some similar points with the descriptions in the Synoptic Gospels and another place where the important element of *performing* healing appears:

- *And a great multitude was following Him, because they were seeing the signs...*

Christ was able to attract a multitude due to the healing and miracles in His ministry. The Church will not be able to accomplish the final harvest without this important element of ministry becoming increasingly commonplace in the Church. There is every reason to believe that many more believers will become *equipped* to *perform* healing and miracles as the Church nears the end of the age. The ministry of Christ will be multiplied in the last days in every aspect in the lives of those who believe.

- _the signs which He was performing on those who were sick._

The apostle John supplies a definition of signs in these verses. The _signs_ that John is referring to have to do with ministry to the _sick_. Christ's ministry of healing and miracles are called _performing signs_ by the apostle John in these verses and in the verses to follow.

This is highly significant information. The idea of _performing signs on the sick_ suggests that Christ had an _element of control_ and could _perform_ the ministry of healing the sick at will. The Greek word that appears frequently in these passages and is translated _performing miracles and healing_ could as easily be translated as _doing miracles and healing_. Christ and His disciples _did_ miracles and healing. This is completely _opposite_ from the idea that healing ministry is unpredictable, unreliable and mysterious. This is an unusual idea for many who have been affected by common misconceptions that healing ministry requires great spirituality and is unpredictable and mysterious. Obviously, healing ministry was predictable, reliable and understood if Christ could _perform signs on the sick_.

The idea of _performing healing_ will also appear in the lives of Christ's disciples in a future chapter. The hope of the author of this book is that every reader will attempt to _perform healing ministry_ after reading the details of this book about *how* this is accomplished. The foundation of being able to consistently *perform healing* is first to be convinced completely that the will of the Father is revealed in Christ's example. Of course, this is precisely why this text is exhaustively examining Christ concerning this matter.

John's Second General Description

John's Gospel, Chapter 7 reveals the reaction of people to the signs in Christ's ministry as well. Many believed that He was the Christ because of the miracles and healing. This is the sixteenth general description of Christ's healing ministry.

> *But many of the multitude believed in Him; and they were saying, "When the Christ shall come, He will not perform more signs than those which this man has, will He?" John 7:31*

The idea of *performing signs* is prominent in these passages. These are important points to consider and review:

- *But many of the multitude believed in Him...*

Again, *many of the multitude* believed that Jesus was the Christ because of the visible miracles and healing in His ministry. *Why should it be any different today?* Without this capacity, the Church will be unequipped to finish the harvest. Technique and polish are not the answer.

Believers must be equipped supernaturally to reach the multitudes.

- *and they were saying, "When the Christ shall come, He will not perform more signs than those which this man has, will He?*

Again, the apostle John describes visible healing and miracle ministry of Christ as *performing signs*. Apparently, Christ had *performed* a large number of *signs* in their presence in order to get this kind of public reaction. They could not conceive of anyone *performing more signs* than Jesus did.

John's Third General Description

The third passage in the Gospel of John also sadly reveals that some did not believe even though they had seen a large number of healing and miracles. This is the seventeenth general description of Christ's healing ministry to the masses found in the Gospels.

> *But though He had performed so many signs before them, yet they were not believing in Him...*
> *John 12: 37*

This general description has a negative tone to it. However, it reveals additional information that confirms the realities of the experience of healing ministry.

- *But though He had performed so many signs before them...*

Christ's Ministry to the Masses
in Luke, John and Acts

This is the third time that miracle and healing ministry is described as *performing signs* by the apostle John. In this case, John reveals that Christ had performed *many* signs.

- *...yet they were not believing in Him...*

Unfortunately, for some in that day, as today, miracles and healing were not enough to bring them to faith in Christ. Unbelieving opposition is always present. Miracle and healing ministry will nearly always find opposition among the unequipped religious establishment. Those who fail to become equipped in the miraculous as the age progresses to its end may find themselves tempted to become critics of those who become equipped to supernaturally help the ill and injured.

John's Fourth General Description

The final description of Christ's healing ministry in the Gospel of John is found in the book's final verses and is the eighteenth general description found in the four Gospels.

> *Many other signs therefore Jesus also performed in the presence of the disciples, which are not written in this book; but these have been written that you may believe that Jesus is the Christ, the Son of God; and that believing you may have life in His name. John 20:30-31*

Performing Miracles and Healing

Anyone carefully, honestly and logically considering all these passages should become convinced that _performing healing and miracles_ as _signs_ is an important aspect of the ministry of Christ. In fact, the passage reveals Christ _performed many other signs_ that are not recorded. In other words, Christ performed many other healings and miracles that cannot be examined. Those events that were selected by the writers of the New Testament were selected because they offer something special about these matters beyond the ordinary events of healing and miracles. Those specific events that the writers chose to record will be reviewed in future chapters.

- _Many other signs therefore Jesus also performed in the presence of the disciples, which are not written in this book..._

Many miracles and healing were _performed_ by Christ that are _not recorded_ in the Gospel of John. By implication, most of these events are not recorded by the other Gospel writers either. This is because the other three Gospels were written _before_ the Gospel of John, and it is very likely that John was familiar with the other three Gospels when this statement was recorded.

- _...but these have been written that you may believe that Jesus is the Christ, the Son of God; and that believing you may have life in His name_

John reveals his purpose in recording the miracles and healing ministry of Jesus Christ. John wants his readers to believe because of these events. Some are critical of those who think that healing and miracle ministry is important. In some cases, these critics have suggested that those who place some emphasis on these miraculous events are being carnal. This would, of course, place the Savior, the Twelve apostles, Paul and many others in the category of the carnal. Obviously, the Apostle John would not agree with these modern critics. More than 100 years old, and after more than 70 years of reflection on Christ's ministry, the apostle John places great emphasis on the miracles and healing of Christ. These are the very last words written to be included in the Canon of Scripture and these words place an emphasis on the miraculous works of Christ.

General Descriptions in the Book of Acts

The final group of passages that describe in a general sense the ministry of Jesus Christ to the masses are found in the book of Acts. The first of these passages is found in Acts Chapter 2. These are the recorded words of the apostle Peter after the outpouring of the Holy Spirit on the day of Pentecost. His general description of the ministry of the Savior is wonderful!

> *Men of Israel, listen to these words: Jesus the Nazarene, a man attested to you by God with miracles and wonders and signs which God performed through Him in your midst, just as you yourselves know... Acts 2:22*

There are some important points to draw from this description from Peter recorded by Luke:

Performing Miracles and Healing

- *...Jesus the Nazarene, a man...*

Some seem to forget that Christ is truly example to believers in all matters. Christ can only be the example if He was a real man. Christ must be seen as *fully human* without denial that He was *fully God*. This is the foundational biblical truth of the Incarnation of Jesus Christ. Here Peter reminds that Jesus was from Nazareth and was a real man. Without recognition of this biblical fact of Christ's humanity, no one can expect to do the *greater works* that Christ promises.

- *...a man attested to you by God with miracles and wonders and signs...*

God attested to Jesus by the miracles, wonders and signs in His ministry. In a future chapter, this book will review the biblical facts that God *attested* to the ministry of Christ's disciples by the same sort of phenomena. Believers should expect that God would *attest* to His servants today by the same sort of gracious acts of power bringing supernatural help to the sick, injured and afflicted.

- *...signs which God performed through Him...*

Again in this passage, Luke reports that Christ was a man with *God performing* healing and other miraculous acts *through Him*. If believers attribute the miracles and healing in Christ's ministry to His divinity, they will never really understand how His disciples were able to heal like Christ; and how today, believers, as His disciples, are able to heal the sick. Christ, despite His divinity, was _a man being used by the Father_ to heal the sick while on earth. The divine balance in healing and miracle ministry is revealed here. Jesus performed the healing and miracles as God did them through Him.

- _...God performed through Him in your midst, just as you yourselves know..._

Even His enemies, most who were religious, were eyewitnesses to the miracles and healing in His ministry. However, this attestation by God was not enough for them. They still chose not to believe. Miracles and healing, therefore, should produce faith in Christ. However, faith was not always the result then and is not always the result today. Some Christians today have been taught _not to believe_ despite Christ's example and teaching. The uninstructed masses, however, will come to Christ in great numbers when His Church demonstrates His power at the end of the age.

This was the nineteenth general description of the supernatural ministry of Christ to the masses found in the New Testament. The twentieth general description is found in Acts, Chapter 10.

The Final General Description
The final verse that reveals something in a general way about the ministry of Christ is found in Acts Chapter 10. In this passage, the apostle Peter is preaching the

Gospel to the Roman Centurion, Cornelius, and his family. Peter describes the Savior in this fashion:

> *You know of Jesus of Nazareth, how God anointed Him with the Holy Spirit and with power, and how He went about doing good, and healing all who were oppressed by the devil; for God was with Him. Acts 10:38*

This concluding passage is perhaps the most general description of the ministry of Christ that has been expressed. Many of the other descriptions were of events in a single season or particular location in Christ's earthly mission. Here the description is of the entire ministry of Christ from start to finish. From this short passage, a wealth of information is obtained:

- *...Jesus of Nazareth...*

Again, Christ was a man from a particular town. *Understanding that Christ ministered miraculously as a human being is exceedingly important to the foundation of any healing ministry.* The Holy Spirit uses real people with all their flaws, failures and forgiven sins.

- *...how God anointed Him with the Holy Spirit...*

Christ was *anointed*, not with oil as the Old Testament anointed ones, but with the Holy Spirit. When John the Baptist, baptized Him in water, the Holy Spirit descended upon Him. The Holy Spirit empowered and guided Him to perform the will of the Father. In similar fashion, Holy Spirit empowers believers to do the will of the Father today. Getting anointed by the Spirit for service is important but is not the only issue. Too many _already_ anointed believers are _passively waiting_ for the Father to reveal things that He has _already revealed_ in His Son. Consequently, they fail to operate in faith in healing and miracles.

- _...and with power..._

Jesus was anointed not only with the Holy Spirit but with _power_. There is an obvious connection throughout the New Testament between _the Holy Spirit_ and _power_[2]. In this case, the _power_ mentioned here is _to do good_ and _to heal all that were oppressed of the devil._

- _...and how He went about doing good..._

Should a person desire an example of what the Father considers as _good_, all is needed is a study of the life of Christ. Any other attitude or teaching concerning healing that is not revealed in Christ's behavior, teaching and attitudes cannot be considered _doing good._

- _...and healing all..._

The apostle Peter like the Gospel writers reveals that Christ _healed all_. The term _healing_ in this general description is obviously describing the undoing of the devil's work. In this case, _healing_ is apparently being used

---

[2] For example, Acts 1:8.

as a general term to describe all the kinds of supernatural ministry that Christ conducted that brought deliverance and healing to people who came to Him.

- *...all who were oppressed by the devil*

The Greek word that is translated *oppressed* is *katadunasteuo.* This word means:

> *...to overpower or exercise hard control over someone; to use power against someone; to tyrannize over someone; to dominate or exploit someone.*[3]

This is what *Christ's healing* is overcoming; *the devil's power to tyrannize and control a person with pain, sickness and disease.* This is simple and wonderfully profound. The Father does not want sickness, injury and pain to control His children. Greater than any good human father, the Father wants the best for His children.

- *...for God was with Him...*

This again places an emphasis on the fact that Christ was not doing His own will but the will of the Father. Christ was not using His own divine power but God the Father and the Holy Spirit were at work in Him. Christ in the Scriptures is a man anointed and empowered by the Holy Spirit acting out the will of God the Father on earth.

---

[3] Vines, pg. 815, Bauer, pg. 410

Christ's Ministry to the Masses
in Luke, John and Acts

Summary of the Twenty General Descriptions

Four general descriptions of Christ's ministry to masses of people are found in Matthew's Gospel. Three are found in Mark's Gospel. Seven are identified in Luke's Gospel. Four are found in the Gospel of John. Two more are found in the Acts of the Apostles.

Preaching the Gospel of the Kingdom is mentioned in five of the general descriptions of the healing and miracle ministry of Christ. Reference to casting out demons, demoniacs, or the devil is mentioned in six of the twenty general descriptions.

In the twenty general descriptions revealing Christ's healing ministry to the masses, only one *specifically* addresses the possibility of someone not being healed. In that particular case, Christ Himself reveals the reason. Christ explained that *unbelief* on the part of those in His hometown was the reason that only a few were healed and there were no miracles. The control was not with God the Father but with those in His hometown. They limited what Christ could do by their unbelief.

There is *no suggestion* in any of these accounts that the will of the Father might be different for different people in the matter of healing. Christ *never* hesitates to heal someone in the passages that have been examined. He *already knows* what the will of the Father will be for the thousands of people He healed. In fact, in some of the events, the passages reveal that Christ *healed all* that came to Him in a multitude.

Performing Miracles and Healing

Additionally, the impressive idea of Christ *performing healing and miracles* as *signs* is presented in a number of passages. Along with His powerful supernatural ministry, the important truth of Christ doing these things *as a man,* rather than as God, is revealed.

This brings to a conclusion the consideration of the general descriptions of the ministry of Christ to the masses. Shortly, this book will consider the specific events of Christ healing individuals. However, it is entirely appropriate to first consider the general descriptions found in the New Testament of Christ's followers duplicating His ministry to the masses.

~4~

The Twelve Apostles' Healing Ministry

Evidence seems to be accumulating that much modern theology concerning healing is good intentioned but passive and impotent since it has failed to make Christ the foundation. What should be the role of believers today in healing and miracles? Does the New Testament speak to believers specifically today about these matters? The answer is that Christ does speak concerning the modern believer's role as He speaks to the Twelve apostles. Consider the command of Christ to the Twelve apostles that has been called *the Great Commission*.

And Jesus came up and spoke to them, saying, "All authority has been given to Me in heaven and on earth. Go therefore and make disciples of all the nations, baptizing them in the name of the Father

and the Son and the Holy Spirit, teaching them to observe all that I commanded you; and lo, I am with you always, even to the end of the age."
Matthew 28:18-20

Why this is important to this discussion of the modern believer's responsibilities to the ministry of healing may not be entirely evident from a quick reading of these verses. However, studying what Christ *actually says* yields powerful results. Consider these thoughts:

- *...All authority has been given to Me in heaven and on earth. Go therefore and make disciples...*

Because the Father has granted *all authority* to Christ, He commands believers in the same way as His Father did Him. The Father wishes to *duplicate* the ministry of His Son in all believers. The Father's will is perfectly revealed through Christ's commands to His disciples as well as it has been through His teaching, actions, works and attitudes.

Christians are to *go* and *make disciples* to Christ. It is not enough to make *believers* in Christ. Disciples must make *disciples*. However, they are not really *disciples* if they are not the kind of *believers* that have real faith and work the works of God. Consider the next phrase of Christ's command.

- *...make disciples of all the nations ...teaching them to observe all that I commanded you...*

The Twelve Apostles' Healing Ministry

The first Twelve apostles were commanded by Christ to make disciples. These disciples were to be taught to *observe all things that Christ commanded the Twelve apostles.* Modern believers are often not taught to observe the commands of Christ to the Twelve. This must change. Believers today must take seriously what Christ told His first apostles to do. Fortunately, the four Gospel writers recorded several passages of Christ's commands and His instruction to His apostles. In other words, believers today can read and observe what Christ commanded the Twelve apostles to do and from those instructions *determine what believers today are commanded to do and teach as well.* For example, the apostle Matthew recorded these events of the ministry of Christ.

And Jesus was going about all the cities and the villages, teaching in their synagogues, and proclaiming the Gospel of the Kingdom, and healing every kind of disease and every kind of sickness. Matthew 9:35

This verse is near the end of Chapter 9 of Matthew's Gospel. When this was written, there were no chapter divisions in Matthew's Gospel. Chapter and verse divisions were added for the sake of convenience centuries later. Therefore, the next verses, which are the first verses of Chapter 10 actually continue the context and ideas of Chapter 9.

And having summoned His twelve disciples, He gave them authority over unclean spirits, to cast them out, and to heal every kind of disease and every kind of sickness...These twelve Jesus sent out after instructing

73

them, saying, "Do not go in the way of the Gentiles, and do not enter any city of the Samaritans; but rather go to the lost sheep of the house of Israel. And as you go, preach, saying, 'The Kingdom of heaven is at hand.' Heal the sick, raise the dead, cleanse the lepers, cast out demons; freely you received, freely give..."
Matthew 10:1, 5-8

There are several points in this passage that demand attention and elaboration:

- *He gave them authority over unclean spirits, to cast them out, and to heal every kind of disease and every kind of sickness...*

This is extremely significant. Christ appointed His disciples with the *same kind of ministry* that He Himself had. In Matthew, Chapter 9, verse 35, the text reveals that Jesus was *healing every kind of disease and every kind of sickness*. In other words, the twelve disciples were commissioned to *duplicate* the supernatural ministry of Jesus Christ and do the very same things in healing that Christ had done. The Twelve were to *cast out demons and to heal every kind of disease and every kind of sickness.*

In the Great Commission, Christ commanded these Twelve apostles to a very specific thing. These Twelve apostles were to *make disciples.* These disciples were to be taught to *observe the very same things* that the Twelve apostles were taught concerning supernatural ministry. In other words, every command from Christ to the Twelve apostles applies to every disciple in every generation thereafter. Unfortunately, many modern disciples have not been taught to observe the commands of Christ to the Twelve for themselves. They read these commands in passing and wrongly assume that those commands were only for the Twelve apostles. Christ's words, contained in the Great Commission, say otherwise. These commands are for any disciple of Christ today.

If Christian leaders fail to do and to teach what Christ commanded the Twelve to do, the only alternative is to invent a powerless substitute that will produce ministries that are not similar to Christ's supernatural ministry at all. Today, many ministers pattern themselves after some outwardly successful minister whom they respect. Unfortunately, much of what has been passed down from generation to generation by these respected leaders, now has the deceptive appearance of orthodoxy. Sometimes respected leaders who are Christ-like in many ways have inherited a powerless form of ministry that does not duplicate Christ's supernatural ministry. When this is true, it is nearly certain that those who are discipled by this leader also will assume that powerlessness is normal. These leaders and their disciples may even embrace the various theological forms of cessationism that may explain why New Testament power is not to be expected today and why the Great Commission cannot be obeyed as Christ said it. Other Christ-like leaders can be good examples in some areas of Christian life and ministry, but Christ alone is the pattern. Any theology that removes Christ and His commands from primary focus is a heresy no matter how respected its human source may be.

Performing Miracles and Healing

As the Church proceeds to the end of the age, more ministries will have vision to fulfill the very words of the Great Commission. They will actually teach and practice what Christ commanded His apostles to do. They will send out prepared disciples who will _duplicate_ the ministry of Christ.

- _These twelve Jesus sent out after instructing them..._

It is not enough to be commissioned and sent out, one must be _instructed_ as how supernatural ministry works. _Instruction_ came _before_ sending them. There is a great deal of failure in this aspect of ministry. Many, while divinely commissioned to heal the sick and cast out demons, do not have the theology or practical information about _how_ healing or deliverance ministry actually works in practice.

Many, while believing theoretically in healing, hang on to erroneous ideas about healing and deliverance that may block any consistent ministry to the sick. These erroneous, unscriptural ideas may have the deceptive appearance of orthodoxy. These ministers need to open themselves to _instruction_ from those who can consistently heal and deliver in the name of Jesus. This may require humility for ministries that are already established. That humility, however, will bring greater grace in their ability to help others. Thank God that these things are increasingly happening in this day. The Lord of the Harvest is sending _conformed_ laborers into His harvest. These disciples are _conformed_ to the image of the Lord in character, gifts and pattern of ministry.

76

- _And as you go, preach, saying, 'The Kingdom of heaven is at hand.' Heal the sick, raise the dead, cleanse the lepers, cast out demons..._

The three elements (the _proclamation_ of the Gospel of the Kingdom, _healing_ and _casting out demons_) are all present in this command. Disciples of Christ are to unashamedly preach the same Gospel of the Kingdom and do the same kinds of supernatural works that Christ did in helping people. Again, this reveals that the Holy Spirit is at work creating the image of Jesus Christ in believers. The ministry of Jesus Christ is being _duplicated_ in believers. Every Christian ministry's goal should be to be increasing _in His image_ and increasingly _duplicating_ Christ's ministry.

Two other elements are found here that have not been present in the other general statements about Christ's ministry found in previous chapters. These two elements are _raise the dead_ and _cleanse the lepers_. However, these two elements are present in the specific incidents of Christ's ministry. Christ raised three people from the dead and cleansed a number of lepers. In other words, Christ is commanding that His miraculous ministry be _duplicated_ in every small and large detail.

- _Heal the sick, raise the dead, cleanse the lepers, cast out demons..._

There is no ambivalence in this statement. There is no _double-mindedness_ in Christ's command. Christ assumes that His commissioned and instructed disciples *will be able* to accomplish the same supernatural ministry that He accomplished. The Twelve and those that followed them accomplished Christ's supernatural ministry consistently.

- *...freely you received, freely give...*

What had the Twelve *received* that they had to *give*? In the scriptural context, the next verse deals with money. However, the original Twelve apostles were not wealthy with the possible exception of Judas. They were *working folks*. The Twelve had just received authority to heal and to cast out demons without any cost to them personally. They had healing and deliverance from demons *to give to others without cost*.

Christ assumes here that they will be able to accomplish healing and deliverance at a level that *greed* might become an issue. He commands them to *freely give* what they have *freely received*. Christ assumes a capacity in His disciples to *give away* healing and deliverance from evil spirits to others as a regular, on-going part of their ministry. In other words, Christ is revealing that they have the same capacity to *perform* healing and miracles as He did. Christ's attitude is very different than much modern theology. Much modern theology treats healing and deliverance ministry as if it were an outlandish, curious, and mysterious matter. Often if a theology acknowledges healing and deliverance at all, that teaching treats it as if it only happens incidentally, unpredictably and not regularly in service to Christ. In contrast, Christ expects His followers to follow Him into healing and miracle ministry as a regular aspect of their ministries.

Failure to simply *believe* Christ's words is actually what produces the ineffectiveness of some Christians in the ministry of healing, miracles and deliverance. However, there is an earlier failure that generally produces the failure to believe. That failure is a failure to teach Christ's commands to do the supernatural. Usually some complex teaching is used to explain why believers today cannot do what the early Church did. Failure to *teach* Christ's disciples that they should do these things that Christ commanded in these passages is a serious disobedience to the commands found in the Great Commission.

Another passage revealing the Father's will for Christ's disciples to heal the sick is found in Luke's Gospel. In that passage where Christ sends seventy to preach and heal, He says:

> *Now after this the Lord appointed seventy others, and sent them two and two ahead of Him to every city and place where He Himself was going to come... And He was saying to them, "The harvest is plentiful, but the laborers are few; therefore beseech the Lord of the harvest to send out laborers into His harvest...And whatever city you enter, and they receive you, eat what is set before you; and heal those in it who are sick, and say to them, 'The Kingdom of God has come near to you'."*
> *Luke 10:1, 8-9*

Performing Miracles and Healing

There are some familiar and less familiar things here:

- *...And He was saying to them, "The harvest is plentiful, but the laborers are few; therefore beseech the Lord of the harvest to send out laborers into His harvest..."*

Christ commands the believer to pray that laborers would be sent into the plentiful harvest. In contrast to some modern teaching on prayer for the lost, the harvest must be *already prepared* for reaping if laborers are needed. In another place, Jesus said that the fields are *white with harvest*[1]. A few verses later Christ then explains what these laborers should be doing in the harvest.

- *...and heal those in it (the city where you enter) who are sick...*

Laborers in the harvest will need to be able to *duplicate* the ministry of Christ. They will need to be able to consistently heal the sick and cast out demons. Christ assumes again in this phrase that healing would be an expected, regular expression of Christian ministry.

- *...and say to them, 'The Kingdom of God has come near to you'.*

The Gospel of the Kingdom is also present in this command of Christ. Believers are to be equipped to proclaim the Gospel of the Kingdom of God. Again,

---

[1] John 4:35

healing ministry is *intimately connected* with *preaching* the Gospel of the Kingdom. The ministry of Christ is to be *duplicated* by His disciples in this matter as well as healing and casting out demons.

Modern theological expressions would dispute that believers should expect that the ministry of Christ would be *duplicated* in them. They think that it was true for the Twelve apostles but not for believers today. However, when they dispute that healing ministry is commanded for believers today in the same way that it was for the Twelve apostles, they dispute the words of Christ that believers should be taught to *obey all things that Christ commanded the Twelve*. Of course, they ensure that anyone believing them, rather than the words of Christ, will have a less than Christ-like ministry. Unfortunately, this is extremely detrimental to those who need the healing and deliverance ministry of Christ. Fortunately, there are fewer everyday in the Church that resist the actual words of the Great Commission. The fact is that *everyone* Christ sent *healed* the sick and cast out demons just like He did. The end of the age is near and the Father has ordained great things for the Church as she prepares to meet her Bridegroom. The Bride must learn to be like Her Bridegroom, Christ, in all respects.

The Twelve Apostles Duplicate Christ's Ministry

It is not hard to see that the disciples took the words of Christ seriously in this matter of healing. For instance, consider the prayer of Peter and John after being commanded and threatened by religious authorities not speak any more of Jesus Christ.

"And now, Lord, take note of their threats, and grant that Thy bond-servants may speak Thy word with all confidence, while Thou dost extend Thy hand to heal, and signs and wonders take place through the name of Thy holy servant Jesus." And when they had prayed, the place where they had gathered together was shaken, and they were all filled with the Holy Spirit, and began to speak the word of God with boldness. Acts 4:29-31

These verses show that in the face of resistance, the leadership of the early Church responded with an interesting prayer that revealed what they expected the risen Christ would be willing to do. They were clear on the will of the Father in the matter of healing.

- *"And now, Lord, take note of their threats, and grant that Thy bond-servants may speak Thy word with all confidence..."*

This seems to be a common prayer found in the New Testament. Believers should speak the Word of God with boldness and confidence. This text will consider later *why* boldness is necessary and show the negative effects of failure to proclaim the Gospel boldly and with faith.

- *"...while Thou dost extend Thy hand to heal, and signs and wonders take place through the name of Thy holy servant Jesus."*

Clearly, Peter and John expected that Christ would validate the Gospel with *signs and wonders*. It should not escape the reader that the prayer here says that _signs and wonders_ would take place through the _name of Jesus_. In other words, they prayed that as they preached the Gospel God would heal those they prayed for in the name of Jesus. This suggests that they expected healing and miracles to happen. It suggests they understood that the Gospel would not have the Father's intended effect without healing, signs and wonders. Further, there is no thought in this verse that anything had changed either in the plan or will of God the Father. The Twelve were going to pray for the sick in the name of Jesus, and expected that Christ would heal and deliver through them just as He had done previously in His earthly ministry.

Some who see healing as being an unpredictable, mysterious, sovereign act of God should be instructed by these verses. These verses reveal that the disciples believed God would heal and grant signs and wonders simply because they had prayed in the name of Jesus. They thought of this as a normal expected expression of their ministries.

Additionally, there is nothing in this passage to suggest that the disciples should divide people into categories of those who should be healed and those who should not be healed. They knew God wanted people well, whole and strong and did not seek the will of the Father on this matter. The Twelve apostles _already_ understood the Father's will in this matter by observation of Christ's ministry first hand. There is no hint that the Twelve believed that sickness or injury might be doing someone some mysterious good. They simply asked the Father to do again what He had promised, what He had revealed in His Son, Jesus, and what Christ had commanded them to accomplish. *How did the Father respond to their prayer?*

- *And when they had prayed, the place where they had gathered together was shaken, and they were all filled with the Holy Spirit, and began to speak the word of God with boldness.*

The Father places His unmistakable stamp of approval on this prayer by the outward sign of an earthquake and by an inward sign of filling them with the Holy Spirit again. The Father granted them the boldness and the attesting signs and wonders they had asked for as they spoke the Word of God.

Shortly after this prayer was uttered, the Book of Acts records the results of their preaching the Word of God with boldness.

> *And at the hands of the apostles many signs and wonders were taking place among the people; and they were all with one accord in Solomon's portico. But none of the rest dared to associate with them; however, the people held them in high esteem. And all the more believers in the Lord, multitudes of men and women, were constantly added to their number; to such an extent that they even carried the sick out into the streets, and laid them on cots and pallets, so that when Peter came by, at least his shadow might fall on any one of them. And also the people from the cities in the vicinity of Jerusalem were*

coming together, bringing people who were sick or afflicted with unclean spirits; and they were all being healed. Acts 5:12-16

There are a number of interesting elements in this passage that are pertinent to this discussion.

- _And at the hands of the apostles many signs and wonders were taking place among the people..._

The text reveals that the ministry of Christ continued powerfully through the apostles. Indeed, these miraculous events were happening at the _hands of the apostles._ This statement implies that these events were _not_ sovereign acts of God. These events were at least in partial control of the apostles. The fact that there were _many_ of these _signs and wonders_ opposes and challenges the attitude seen in many churches that the miraculous will be infrequent and mysterious. Obviously, these signs and wonders were not infrequent or mysterious to the apostles and should not be today.

- _...And all the more believers in the Lord, multitudes of men and women, were constantly added to their number..._

The healing, signs and wonders had a powerful and intended effect beyond the obvious help that ill and injured people received. Multitudes became believers in Christ. Supernatural ministry was important in evangelism then, and is still important today. Supernatural ministry creates an atmosphere where faith in Christ becomes infectious and a spiritual momentum for good is obtained.

- *...to such an extent that they even carried the sick out into the streets, and laid them on cots and pallets, so that when Peter came by, at least his shadow might fall on any one of them.*

The behavior of these people reveals that they had great anticipation of healing. The number of healings, signs and wonders created an expectant faith in the people. God showed extravagant grace in response to the growing faith of these people to the extent of some unusual miracles. Some were healed by simply having Peter's shadow cross them. This is similar to those who were healed by simply touching Christ's clothing, sometimes without His foreknowledge.

Healing a number of the sick through the unusual means of Peter's shadow is revealing. It reveals that *no matter how* these people responded in faith to Christ, the Father would heal them. The expectant faith of the people was the essential element in healing and the healing was not some sort of unexplainable, unpredictable, or sovereign act of God.

- *...And also the people from the cities in the vicinity of Jerusalem were coming together, bringing people who were sick or afflicted with unclean spirits; and they were all being healed.*

This is strongly reminiscent of Christ's ministry, as it should be. The Twelve were _duplicating_ the ministry of Christ. Additionally, again _all were being healed._ Luke also uses the word _healed_ to describe ministry to those who had unclean spirits as well as to those who were sick. This may imply that the unclean spirits were causing sickness as well as other problems. However, this does not suggest that evil spirits cause all sickness.

Summary of the Twelve Apostle's Ministry
The general descriptions of the ministry of Christ's followers reveal a number of important points which are not new to the readers of this book:

- The bold proclamation of the Gospel and the miraculous are found together repeatedly. This is like the ministry of Christ.

- Healing and casting out demons are often found together. This is like the ministry of Christ as well.

- The idea of _performing miracles_ is repeatedly found in various passages describing the ministry of the Twelve. This reveals that the _performer_ must know _how_ to perform miracles. This expression, _performing miracles_, is also found repeatedly in the Gospel of John accounts concerning Christ's ministry.

- The general accounts occasionally reveal that _all_ were healed in a situation concerning the ministry of the followers of Christ. However, these accounts are more likely not to address how many were healed in any situation.

- These general accounts *never* describe anyone *not* being healed as a result of God's will. This is also like the ministry of Christ. Therefore, those who express the idea that it might not be God's will to heal someone are expressing a theological idea that has *not been found at all* in the general descriptions of the ministry of Christ or His Twelve apostles.

~5~

Ministry to the Masses by Stephen, Philip, Barnabus & Paul

General Descriptions of Stephen and Philip

In the Book of Acts there is a short description of the supernatural ministry of Stephen in language that is strongly reminiscent of the descriptions of the Lord Jesus Christ in the Gospel of John. Stephen was one of the first seven deacons of the Church, and had the distinction of being the first martyr of the Church. For a short time until his death, Stephen was *duplicating* the ministry of Christ in *performing wonders and signs.*

> *And Stephen, full of grace and power, was performing great wonders and signs among the people. Acts 6:8*

The fact that Stephen was able to *perform signs* is striking. Again, the miraculous certainly was not mysterious to Stephen. Stephen understood *how* to *perform signs*. Stephen knew that the Holy Spirit would cooperate with him in miracle ministry as He had done with Christ and the Twelve apostles.

Philip, the First Evangelist

Another one of the original seven deacons also reveals the ministry of Christ in a spectacular way. The Book of Acts in another place tells us that this man, Philip, was an evangelist. In fact, Philip is the *only* evangelist that the New Testament tells us about. Fortunately, this passage gives us much more detail about the ministry of Philip than the passage concerning Stephen.

> *And Philip went down to the city of Samaria and began proclaiming Christ to them. And the multitudes with one accord were giving attention to what was said by Philip, as they heard and saw the signs which he was performing. For in the case of many who had unclean spirits, they were coming out of them shouting with a loud voice; and many who had been paralyzed and lame were healed. And there was much rejoicing in that city.... And even Simon himself believed; and after being baptized, he continued on with Philip; and as he observed signs*

and great miracles taking place, he was constantly amazed. Acts 8:5-8, 13

Philip reveals many of the same points that have been found in passages concerning Christ in the Gospels. Philip was *duplicating* the ministry of Christ.

- *And Philip went down to the city of Samaria and began proclaiming Christ to them.*

In previous passages, Christ proclaimed the Kingdom of God. In this case, the King, Jesus Christ, is being proclaimed. This is another expression of the Gospel of the Kingdom. Additionally, in the next phase, the same *triad* of elements is found again; *the proclamation of Gospel, healing and deliverance from evil spirits.* Anything less than this kind of experience will be somewhat less than a New Testament experience of ministry.

- *And the multitudes with one accord were giving attention to what was said by Philip, as they heard and saw the signs which he was performing.*

Philip, like Christ before him, had the attention of the multitudes because of the *signs* that he was *performing.* Philip was able to *perform these signs.* This seriously questions the idea that healing and miracles are mysterious sovereign acts of God. Obviously, these things were not very mysterious to Philip. He knew *how* to *perform* them just as Christ and the Twelve apostles and Stephen understood *how* to *perform* them. The next phrase to consider reveals what these *signs* were exactly. This phrase reveals what a biblical New Testament *sign* is.

- *For in the case of many who had unclean spirits, they were coming out of them shouting with a loud voice; and many who had been paralyzed and lame were healed.*

The two kinds of supernatural ministry that are revealed here as *signs* are *casting out demons* and *healing*. In particular, the paralyzed and lame are pointed out as being healed. *Many* were healed and *many* were delivered from unclean spirits. The New Testament repeatedly reveals these two aspects of supernatural ministry together.

The Gospels and Acts of the Apostles do *not* draw strong distinctions between healing and deliverance from evil spirits. Healing is treated much like deliverance from evil spirits by the authors of the New Testament. The same attitudes seem to be expressed by the writers of Scripture toward both aspects of ministry. This strongly suggests that illness and injury are the same sort of enemies to humanity that evil spirits are. Christ, the Twelve apostles, Stephen and Philip all treat demons and sickness in the same manner. They *never* say or suggest by their behavior that sickness or injury might be a friend at times. Their behavior toward sickness is *just like* their behavior toward demons.

- *And there was much rejoicing in that city...*

Ministry to the Masses by Stephen, Philip, Barnabus and Paul

Preaching of the gospel and Christ's supernatural ministry through His servants will transform lives by delivering them from afflictions of the devil, sickness, disease and debilitating conditions. Anyone with normal logic should see that this would produce rejoicing in proportion to the number of people experiencing release and relief.

On the other hand, religious teaching suggests that believers ought to rejoice in a mysterious work of God being done in the pain and disabling work of continuing sickness and disease. In fact, often these same people will logically seek healing from a physician because they *know intuitively* that disabling sickness and pain are not really blessings. They would not wish serious pain and suffering upon their own children but somehow think that the Father sees suffering and pain differently than they do. They need to look the true revelation of the Father, Christ Himself, as He consistently reveals the Father's love for His children by healing them.

- *...and even Simon himself believed; and after being baptized, he continued on with Philip; and as he observed signs and great miracles taking place, he was constantly amazed.*

The text tells us that Simon was a prominent magician in the region. Perhaps, Simon was an occultist operating by the power of evil spirits or simply a clever illusionist. The text is not entirely clear on the nature of Simon's magic. However, after observing Philip performing signs and miracles, Simon became a believer and then traveled with Philip to continue to observe the amazing supernatural phenomena in Philip's ministry.

If Simon had had the opportunity to observe the Lord Jesus Christ, he doubtless would have reacted in the same way. While the text tells us that Simon had very serious character problems, he also became an unusually perceptive witness of these events that could have revealed any trickery that was taking place.

- *Absent from the account:* As in many other passages, there is no revelation that some were not healed. While the accounts do not directly state that all were healed, the passages in no way indicate that it might be the will of the Father that some are to remain sick or afflicted by evil spirits.

Paul and Barnabus *Duplicated* Christ's Ministry

Paul and Barnabus also *duplicated* the ministry of Christ in similar fashion as the Twelve apostles and the deacons Stephen and Philip. Shortly after being sent forth by the Holy Spirit from the Church at Antioch, Paul and Barnabus were ministering in Iconium.

And it came about that in Iconium they entered the synagogue of the Jews together, and spoke in such a manner that a great multitude believed, both of Jews and of Greeks. But the Jews who disbelieved stirred up the minds of the Gentiles, and embittered them against the brethren. Therefore they (Paul and Barnabus) spent a long time there speaking boldly with reliance upon the Lord, who was bearing witness to the word of His grace, granting that signs and wonders be done by their hands. Acts 14:1-3

There are several points that should be considered in this passage. This passage is noteworthy because it has the same emphasis as other passages that have been previously considered.

- *Therefore they (Paul and Barnabus) spent a long time there (Iconium) speaking boldly...*

While this passage doesn't say specifically what Paul and Barnabus were speaking, the context reveals that they were certainly speaking about Christ. It is probable that they were preaching the Gospel of the Kingdom of God. Paul and Barnabus were *speaking boldly. Speaking boldly* is a prerequisite for the miraculous. *Why boldness is necessary* is considered in a subsequent chapter.

- *...with reliance upon the Lord who was bearing witness to the word of His grace, granting that signs and wonders be done by their hands.*

In this verse, *the divine balance* can be seen. On the human side of the equation, Barnabus and Paul who were *relying on the Lord.* This reveals the faith of Barnabus and Paul in the Risen Christ.

The divine side of the healing equation was the Risen Christ who was *bearing witness to the word of His grace.* On the human side of the equation, Paul and Barnabus were *boldly* preaching *the word of His grace.* On the divine side of the equation, the risen Christ was bearing witness by *granting that signs and wonders be done by their hands.* On the human side of the equation, Paul and Barnabus' hands were *performing* the *signs and wonders.*

A chapter later in the Book of Acts, the same divine balance in the miraculous is revealed in a report Paul and Barnabus gave to the leaders in Jerusalem.

> *And all the multitude kept silent, and they (the Church leaders in Jerusalem) were listening to Barnabas and Paul as they were relating what signs and wonders God had done through them among the Gentiles. Acts 15:12*

This balance is revealed in the fact that the passage says *God did the signs and wonders through them.* God does the miraculous but does it *through* human vessels. Those who want to completely disconnect the power of God from human vessels do it without biblical license. Those who want to emphasize the sovereignty of God in the miraculous do so at the expense of the human side of the equation seen clearly in the New Testament. Consequently, believers will have less than a biblical capacity to deliver and heal the sick and afflicted if they fail to see the human side of the equation.

A similar, but more detailed statement of the apostle Paul is found in his book to the Romans. This general description of Paul's ministry seems to sum up, in many respects, Paul's theology of the miraculous and its relationship with the gospel.

> *For I will not presume to speak of anything except what Christ has accomplished through me, resulting in the obedience of the Gentiles by word and deed, in the power of signs and wonders, in the power of the Spirit; so that from Jerusalem and round about as far as Illyricum I have fully preached the gospel of Christ. Romans 15:18-19*

The apostle Paul discloses a number of interesting aspects to *duplicating* the ministry of Christ. Paul's lack of hesitation to discuss the miracles, signs and wonders in his ministry is revealing. Today, many would criticize someone who was willing to do this. Modern attitudes towards healing and miracles often are in conflict with biblical values.

- *...what Christ has accomplished through me...*

This is similar to the previous passage about Paul and Barnabus. The divine balance of *Christ working through us* is revealed again.

- *...resulting in the obedience of the Gentiles by word and deed...*

The result of Christ working through Paul was the fruit of ministry among the Gentiles. Many Gentiles had become Christ's disciples measured by the fact that they were obeying His commands given to His apostles. The message Paul was preaching is not mentioned specifically; but since _obedience_ to Christ was its result, it is easy to speculate that the message was the Gospel of the Kingdom of God that has as its centerpiece, the truth of _obedience_ to the Lordship of Christ.

- _...in the power of signs and wonders, in the power of the Spirit..._

Paul reveals what brought about the obedience of the Gentiles to Christ. The miraculous power of the Holy Spirit was responsible for Paul's success. This was due in large part because of signs and wonders that validated the Gospel Paul was preaching.

- _...so that from Jerusalem and round about as far as Illyricum I have fully preached the gospel of Christ..._

Paul explains that to _fully preach the gospel of Christ_ it is necessary to have signs and wonders. Paul understood that _the power of signs and wonders_ validating the gospel was the only way to _fully preach the gospel_ and to bring the maximum number of the Gentiles to _obedience_ to Christ. Repeatedly in this study, there has been a biblical connection between the gospel and the miraculous. Laborers in the harvest must be equipped to preach the Gospel with signs following. The size of the mission of the last days Church will demand that believers know what Paul knew about the Gospel and its relationship with the miraculous.

Ministry to the Masses by
Stephen, Philip, Barnabus and Paul

The apostle Paul also reveals that his apostleship was affirmed by the miraculous validation of his ministry. He says this in his letter that has been called Second Corinthians.

The signs of a true apostle were performed among you with all perseverance, by signs and wonders and miracles. 2 Corinthians 12:12

Paul in the above general description of his ministry, *performed* signs, wonders and miracles. Paul obviously did not think that these things were mysterious. He knew how to *perform signs, wonders and miracles.* Again, the ministry of Christ is being revealed through Paul.

Additionally, Paul reveals that believers should be able to distinguish a true apostle by the capacity he has for the supernatural ministry of Christ. Some have said that perseverance is the sign of the apostle, however, the grammar of this verse does not allow such an interpretation. Perseverance is wonderful and needs to be found in all Christian ministries, but is not the sign that Paul is writing about. The miraculous is the sign of the true apostle.[1] Perseverance in faith allowed Paul to produce the miraculous signs of an apostle. Alternative explanations are often given as a way of preventing consideration of the powerlessness of some ministries claiming apostleship.

---

[1] A whole chapter is devoted to distinguishing the ministry of the apostle from other ministries in the author's book **The Last Apostles on Earth.**

Performing Miracles and Healing

The power to heal is not limited to the apostle, however. For instance, in another passage that reveals Christ working through His Church, Paul lists the nine gifts of the Holy Spirit. *Gifts of healing* and *effecting of miracles* are found with seven other gifts that the Holy Spirit gives to His people.

> *...and to another gifts of healing by the one Spirit, and to another the effecting of miracles...*
> *I Corinthians 12:9b-10a*

There are several points to consider in these verses.

- *...and to another gifts of healing*

If there are other gifts functioning today in the Church, why should healing be different? Paul does not show that one gift in particular is to be desired above the others. All are available for ministry to and through the Church of Jesus Christ. Those who elevate healing and miracles above the other gifts and see these gifts as somewhat more spiritual or harder to accomplish do so without biblical license. These gifts operate exactly like the others. All these spiritual gifts are gifts of God's grace that operate by faith through love.

- *... and to another the effecting of miracles*

One of these gifts to individuals in the church is the *effecting of miracles*. The phrase *the effecting of miracles* is often translated as *the working of miracles* in many versions. The Greek phrase means literally *working,*

100

effecting or operating works of power. The gift of working miracles is to *work works of power*. The very name of this gift reveals that the recipient of the gift knows *how to work miracles*. This reveals that the gift is certainly not mysterious, unpredictable, or unreliable to the one who has received it to serve others.

The context of the passage reveals God placing His various gifts within the Church. In other words, God is giving supernatural gifts to individuals within the Church to bless and strengthen others. This implies that these gifted people will know how to work these gifts. This list of gifts includes healing and miracles. A few verses later, Paul says that some are appointed in the Church to do miracles and healing in the same way that some are appointed as apostles, prophets or teachers.

> *...God has appointed in the church, first apostles, second prophets, third teachers, then miracles, then gifts of healings... 1 Corinthians 12:28*

This listing of supernatural gifts implies that within the local churches there are those who should have these gifts. In other words, there should be those who are gifted to regularly heal and perform miracles in the local churches today. Unfortunately, in many local church situations there is no context where those who are gifted in this way can *learn how* to *perform* miracles. Thankfully, things are changing. Many churches are now having *Schools of the Holy Spirit* or *Schools of the Prophetic* so that gifted individuals can *learn how* to function in supernatural giftings.

The Final General Description of Christ's Disciples

The last general description of the supernatural ministry of Christ being *duplicated* in the disciples is found in the Book of Hebrews. This passage also reveals some similar truths that have been considered before.

> *...how shall we escape if we neglect so great a salvation? After it (the word) was at the first spoken through the Lord, it was confirmed to us by those who heard, God also bearing witness with them, both by signs and wonders and by various miracles and by gifts of the Holy Spirit according to His own will. Hebrews 2:3-4*

This passage does have some new information to discover as well as confirming some things that we have already considered.

- *...After it (the word) was at the first spoken through the Lord, it was confirmed to us by those who heard...*

The writer of Hebrews relates that the original witnesses of Christ, the twelve apostles and the other witnesses *confirmed* the word of Christ to them. This sounds similar to the command of Christ found in the Great Commission. Christ commanded the Twelve apostles to make disciples and to teach these disciples to observe all that He had commanded the apostles to do. This verse reveals much of the same idea. The original hearers taught the Lord's message, the Gospel of the Kingdom of God, to a new group of disciples. They *bore witness* to what they had heard and seen.

- ...*God also bearing witness with them, both by signs and wonders and by various miracles and by gifts of the Holy Spirit...*

Not only did the original hearers bear witness to the message of Christ, but *God bore witness with them.* In other words, God involved Himself in the process of communication of the message of Christ by validating it to the hearers. How did God validate the message of Christ? God *bore witness both by signs and wonders and by various miracles and by gifts of the Holy Spirit.* The message of Christ and the miraculous are found together again.

- ...*according to His own will.*

God grants the miraculous to validate the gospel of Christ. This is abundantly clear and is an expression of the will of God. It is clear that it is God's will to heal, deliver and bless, particularly in response to the bold proclamation of the Gospel. This brings to a close the general accounts of ministry to the masses through Christ's followers. After a brief introduction, this book will now focus on the specific people that were healed in Christ's ministry to learn more of the Father's will.

Section 2

Specific Incidents of Miracles and Healing in Christ's and His Disciples' Ministries

Introduction to Christ's Specific Healings & Miracles

The Gospel Writers' Selection of Specific Events

Without a doubt, only a small portion of the miracles and healing in Christ's ministry are described in any detail by the four authors of the Gospel accounts. Previously, many of the general accounts of Christ healing the masses were reviewed and it is clear that thousands of people were healed in Christ's earthly ministry. Obviously, the Gospels cannot describe in detail these thousands of healings. The apostle John notes this situation at the end of his Gospel. There John says:

> *And there are also many other things which Jesus did, which if they were written in detail, I suppose that even the world itself would not contain the books which were written. John 21:25*

The apostle John tells his readers that he had a specific reason for choosing the particular miracles and healings that his Gospel reviews. His words about this matter are recorded at the end of his Gospel:

> *Many other signs therefore Jesus also performed in the presence of the disciples, which are not written in this book; but these have been written that you may believe that Jesus is the Christ, the Son of God; and that believing you may have life in His name.*
> *John 21:30-31*

John says this to his readers about *why* he chose to record the particular *signs* that are found in his Gospel:

* *Many other signs therefore Jesus also performed in the presence of the disciples, which are not written in this book.*

Nearly all the healing and miracle events that John records are *not* found in the other three Gospels. Since John was probably familiar with the other three Gospels, perhaps he felt it unnecessary to reproduce the events that the other Gospel writers had included. Since there were many other events that no one had recorded, John selected those events that had particularly inspired his *faith in Christ* to include in his book about Christ.

* *but these have been written that you may believe that Jesus is the Christ, the Son of God; and that believing you may have life in His name.*

John tells his readers that he chose particular healings and miracles because he believed those particular healings and miracles would cause his readers to *believe that Jesus is the Christ.* John's selection of particular miracles and healings was governed by his desire that his Gospel would produce *faith in Christ* in its readers. John must have seen something different in the particular miracles and healing which he included that he thought would particularly help his readers with faith in Christ.

Luke, the physician, the companion of the apostle Paul, writer of the Gospel that bears his name and the Acts of the Apostles, also reveals his reasons for writing his Gospel. In the opening verses of his Gospel, Luke writes:

> *Inasmuch as many have undertaken to compile an account of the things accomplished among us, just as those who from the beginning were eyewitnesses and servants of the word have handed them down to us, it seemed fitting for me as well, having investigated everything carefully from the beginning, to write it out for you in consecutive order, most excellent Theophilus; so that you might know the exact truth about the things you have been taught. Luke 1:1-4*

In these four verses, Luke reveals a great deal about his reasons for writing his Gospel. He also reveals a great deal about the circumstance of his writing. Luke begins by telling his readers that he was aware of other accounts of Christ's life.

- *Inasmuch as many have undertaken to compile an account of the things accomplished among us...*

Luke was obviously aware of other *many* other written accounts that had been *compiled* of Christ's teaching and the miraculous events of His life. Many experts believe Luke was written after Mark's and Matthew's Gospels were written. Therefore, Luke may have been referring to the Gospels of Mark and Matthew or perhaps some other compilations which have not survived to the present time.

- *...just as those who from the beginning were eyewitnesses and servants of the word have handed them down to us...*

Luke reminds his readers that these accounts were *compiled* by *eyewitnesses* and *handed down* to those who are not necessarily eyewitnesses of all the events recorded. Of course, Matthew, who was one of the Twelve apostles, would be an excellent *eyewitness* of the events recorded in his Gospel.

- *...it seemed fitting for me as well, having investigated everything carefully from the beginning to write it out for you in consecutive order...*

Luke apparently felt that another Gospel that gave careful attention to *everything* in all the materials he had *investigated* was needed. Luke related these materials in a detailed, *consecutive,* historical account. Luke's Gospel seems to offer additional details that the other Gospels might not. Luke's accounts of specific miracles are often longer than those same miracles found in the other Gospels. He also offers three miracles and several parables that the other Gospel writers do not include at all. Luke also has a great amount of detail about the events surrounding the birth of John the Baptist and the birth of Christ that the other Gospel writers do not include in their accounts.

- *... most excellent Theophilus...*

Luke has addressed this Gospel and the Acts of the Apostles to someone named *Theophilus*. While *Theophilus* was a common name in the First Century, this does not necessarily mean that there was an actual person that Luke was addressing. The name's meaning in Greek is *Lover of God.* Therefore, Luke might have been using this common name to affectionately address all his potential readers as *Lovers of God.* Luke now reveals his real motive for his Gospel.

- *...so that you might know the exact truth about the things you have been taught. Luke 1:1-4*

Luke wants his readers to know the *exact truth* about what Jesus Christ revealed by His life, teaching, death and resurrection.

Both the apostle John and the physician Luke believe that study of their Gospels will have a positive effect on their readers. John believes *faith in Christ* will be the result of reading his Gospel. Luke believes his readers will know the *truth about Christ* when they study his Gospel. Unfortunately, neither Mark nor Matthew reveals to their readers their motivations for writing their Gospels. However, logic suggests their motives were similar. These Gospel writers wanted to reveal *the true Christ* so their readers would *believe in Him*.

There are only twenty-five specific healings or healing miracles performed by Christ recorded in the Gospels. The Gospel writers had specific reasons for selection of the particular miracles and healings each described. There were thousands of miraculous events for each writer to select from.

At the time of the writing of the Gospels, with the exception of the Gospel of John, there were many eyewitnesses alive. Most of the actual people who were healed were still alive to consult with. With all the potential testimonies about Christ, the selection of particular miracles and healings must have been guided by the specific insights the particular account offers. In other words, something special is revealed in each specific event the Gospel's record.

Something unusual is found in those miracles and healings that captured the attention of the writer above the thousands of other healings and miracles. Often the Gospel writers reveal within the accounts *why* a particular unusual miracle took place. Studying these specific accounts reveal principles of healing and miracles that the Gospel writers wanted their readers to understand in order to *duplicate* the ministry of Christ. Truths about faith in Christ as Healer and how healing and miracles work are discerned as these accounts are studied in their detail. Therefore, the next chapters in this book will seek to discern these principles as Christ's ministry of healing is carefully observed.

The Nature of the Synoptic Gospels

There is a great wealth of information in the Gospels regarding the specific teachings and actions of Christ concerning healing. It would be nearly impossible to present if it were not for the unique nature of three of the four Gospels.

Because the Gospels of Matthew, Mark and Luke have a clear relationship between them, they have been called the *Synoptic Gospels.* The term *Synoptic* means *seen together.* These gospels have a striking repetition of events and even exact descriptions. When analyzed and compared, many of the verses in each Synoptic Gospel are *exactly* the same and many other verses are nearly the same. For example, the Gospel of Mark has 661 verses and Matthew's Gospel has 1068 verses. Of Matthew's 1068 verses, 606 of them are either very similar or *exactly* the same as Mark's 661 verses. In fact, of these 606 verses found in Matthew that are similar with Mark's Gospel, 51% are *exactly* the same.

The Gospel of Luke's relationship with Mark's Gospel is similar. Of the Gospel of Luke's 1149 verses, 320 of them are either *exactly* the same or very similar to the Gospel of Mark's 661 verses. Of these 320 verses, 53%

are *exactly* the same. What this means for our study in this book is that each parallel account of a healing and miracle in the Synoptic Gospels does not need to be reviewed in the text where there is exact or near exact repetition. Where there is additional information on the healing or the miracle supplied by the Gospel writer, additional comment will be made when this additional information appears to be pertinent. For example, out of the twenty-five detailed specific healings or healing miracles recorded from the life of Christ, eleven of these events are repeated in all three Synoptic Gospels. What this means is that there are thirty-three parallel passages that cover eleven separate events in the life of Christ. Therefore, it is unnecessary to review twenty-two of these parallel passages in this text except where an account offers additional pertinent information. Two more healing or miracle events are repeated in two Gospels. This means that there are two more parallel accounts that it is unnecessary to review. Twelve healing and miracle events are recorded in only one Gospel. Each of these twenty-five healing and healing miracle events has been reviewed in the chapters to follow.

Some of the miracles in the life of Christ are not included in this book simply because those miracles did not specifically involve a healing. There are miracles that reveal Christ's power over demons, finances, or nature that are not covered in the chapters to follow simply because this book is about healing and healing miracle ministry. Study of these events is worthwhile but will not be conducted in this text.

Introduction to Christ's Specific Healings and Miracles

The chapters to follow are organized around certain healing themes. For instance, nearly all the events where Christ heals a blind person are found in a single chapter. Nearly all the accounts of a healing of a medical condition where the text reveals that the condition was caused by demonic activity are found in the same chapter. A few events could be included in two separate chapters. For example, Christ might heal a blind person by casting out a demon. When encountering an event like this, a decision was made to include the event in a particular chapter but not both chapters.

~6~

Christ Heals the Blind

Two Blind Men Healed by Christ

Early in Christ's ministry, between the time Christ gave the Sermon on the Mount and when He sent the Twelve disciples out to minister, He healed two blind men. This passage, found in Matthew's Gospel Chapter 9, reveals powerful truths concerning healing. It may be even clearer on the matter of who is in control of healing, and concerns two blind men who sought out Christ persistently for healing.

And as Jesus passed on from there, two blind men followed Him, crying out, and saying, "Have mercy on us, Son of David!" And after He had come into the house, the blind men came up to Him, and Jesus said to them, "Do you believe that I am able to do this?" They said to Him, "Yes, Lord." Then He touched their eyes, saying, "Be it done to you according to your faith." And their eyes were opened. And Jesus sternly warned them, saying, " See here, let no one know about this! " But they went out, and spread the news about Him in all that land. Matthew 9:27-31

Consider these points in this passage:

- *And as Jesus passed on from there, two blind men followed Him, crying out, and saying, "Have mercy on us, Son of David!"*

In the normal course of travel from one place to another in ministry, Christ encountered these two blind men. They cried out asking for *mercy*. *Mercy* has a definite meaning. The Greek word for *mercy* in this passage is the verb *eleeo*, which is akin to the noun *eleos*. Vine's Expository Dictionary of New Testament Words says this of *eleos*:

> *It is the outward manifestation of pity; it assumes need on the part of him who receives it and resources adequate to meet the need on the part of him who shows it.*[1]

By asking Christ for *mercy*, these two men demonstrated that they believed Christ had *resources adequate to meet the need*. These two men also identified Christ as the Jewish Messiah by calling Him by the messianic title, *Son of David*. In other words, these two blind men *believed* that Jesus was *the awaited Messiah* and that He had *resources available* to heal their blindness.

---

[1] Vines, pg. 732-3

Christ Heals the Blind

- *And after He had come into the house...*

Apparently, Christ postponed ministry to these men until He had arrived at the house mentioned above. So these two blind men must have followed along after Christ. This kind of travel had to be difficult for these blind men. The fact that they did not give up and made the journey reveals their determination to be healed. It is possible that Christ purposely waited until arriving at the house mentioned above to heal these men. In any case, these men were actively seeking Christ for healing, and Christ was *not* actively seeking them to heal them. They were *initiating* this discourse with Christ concerning their healing. After these two blind men came up to Christ, Christ asked these men an important question.

- *...the blind men came up to Him, and Jesus said to them, "Do you believe that I am able to do this?"*

Believing is the issue. Christ's reaction to these blind men reveals that their *faith* was the central issue in their healing.[2] Christ asks these men if they *believe* He is able to do this. Christ does not ask them about their desperation, their hopes or their sincerity. None of these things are the issue. Faith alone is the issue in their healing.

- *They said to Him, "Yes, Lord." Then He touched their eyes...*

---

[2] The Greek words for *believe* and *faith* come from the same Greek root word. In this case, *Faith* is a noun and *believe* is a verb. These words express essentially the same thing. *To believe* is to *have faith* and to *have faith* is *to believe.*

These two blind men answer that they do _believe_ that Christ can heal them. Their answer also reflects a submissive attitude in that they call Christ _Lord_ meaning _ruler_ or _king_. In response to their _faith_, Christ uses His most ordinary method of imparting healing; He touches their eyes and says:

- _...saying, "Be it done to you according to your faith."_

Christ's earlier question to the men about _believing_ becomes all the more significant now in this verse. This is the second time that Christ has mentioned _faith_ or _believing_ before He heals these men. It is noteworthy that there is no prayer to the Father concerning this matter. Christ already knows the will of the Father in matters of healing. The Father wants people well.

The issue of these men being healed is not a issue of the will of the Father, it is a issue of their faith. In fact, Christ reveals that these two blind men are _in control_ of the matter of their healing. These men will receive from the Father _according to their faith_. They will receive according to their _faith in Christ as Healer_. This implies that they would not have received healing if they had not believed despite what the Father wanted for them.

If the Father wanted to demonstrate that His will is different in the matter of healing for different people, this would have been a great situation to demonstrate it. The Father could have forever established the principle that His will is mysterious in the matter of healing and that He treats different people differently. However, that is not the case in this situation or any other like it in Scripture. Here are two men with the *same* condition of blindness. They seek Christ in the *same* way. Christ asks them the *same* question. They express faith in answering Christ in the *same* way. They are healed in the *same* way. Christ explains their healing in the *same* way.

The healing of both men in the *same* way reveals another biblical principle. *God is not a respecter of persons.* What the Father will do for one person, He will do for another *if* that person meets the *same* conditions. While many have understood this principle when considering other matters such as forgiveness of sins, they have not consistently applied this principle to all aspects of Divine-human interactions.

- *And their eyes were opened...*

These men had precipitated their healings by expressing *faith* through seeking Christ for healing. They had also confessed their *faith* on Christ's questioning of them. Finally, Christ said that they would receive *according to their faith.* They apparently had the *faith* that was needed because their eyes were opened.

The Blind Beggar Bartimaeus' Healing

This account of a miracle is similar to the account of a pair of miracles that was just discussed in this chapter. In that event, which happened chronologically in the first year of Christ's ministry, found in Matthew 9:27-31, Christ healed two blind men. The healing of the blind beggar Bartimaeus happened much later in Christ's ministry. It is near the end of the third year of His ministry. In fact, this is the last healing recorded by Mark, and is just before Christ enters Jerusalem for the last time. This same healing is recorded in Luke 18:35-43, also close to the time that Christ enters Jerusalem. The only significant difference between the accounts is that Luke does not use Bartimaeus' name. Here is the first part of Mark's account:

> *And they came to Jericho. And as He was going out from Jericho with His disciples and a great multitude, a blind beggar named Bartimaeus, the son of Timaeus, was sitting by the road. And when he heard that it was Jesus the Nazarene, he began to cry out and say, "Jesus, Son of David, have mercy on me!" And many were sternly telling him to be quiet, but he kept crying out all the more, "Son of David, have mercy on me!" Mark 10:46-48*

It is entirely possible, even probable, that Bartimaeus had heard about the healing of the two blind men more than two years earlier and reacted logically to this set of events. Bartimaeus could have said to himself. *If God healed them, why not me?* Every person in need should come to that same conclusion and allow the faith and success of others to affect them. God is not a respecter of persons. The people being healed in these situations were entirely normal people. *Whatever the Father has done for them through Christ, He is willing to do for all.*

The words, actions and attitudes of Christ again reveal that the will of the Father is settled in matters of healing. The Father wants people well. Christ reveals the

Christ Heals the Blind

Father in all matters including healing. Here is the beginning of the story:

- *...And as He was going out from Jericho with His disciples and a great multitude, a blind beggar named Bartimaeus, the son of Timaeus, was sitting by the road.*

Earlier in this chapter, the healing of two blind men by Christ was reviewed. These two blind men were not specifically identified by name in the text. In contrast, this account is very specific. It even contains detailed personal information concerning the blind man who was healed. Perhaps Matthew is subtly informing his readers that they could meet the man healed in this story; Bartimaeus, the son of Timaeus who lives near Jericho. Perhaps Matthew is saying to his readers that they can hear about Christ from Bartimaeus if they wish.

- *And when he heard that it was Jesus the Nazarene, he began to cry out and say, "Jesus, Son of David, have mercy on me!" And many were sternly telling him to be quiet, but he kept crying out all the more, "Son of David, have mercy on me!"*

This response of Bartimaeus to the presence of Christ is very similar to the two blind men who were healed. In fact, it is nearly identical. Bartimaeus *cries out*, identifies Christ as *the Son of David* and asks for *mercy*. All these elements in this story are identical to the actions of the two blind men.

Bartimaeus may have thought that since Christ had healed the other two blind men, he might try to *duplicate* as much as possible what he had heard of the healing of the two blind men by saying the same words to Christ. Bartimaeus might have thought that *if Christ healed them on this basis, He will heal me on the same basis.* Up to this point, the actions of the blind men are nearly identical in both stories.

However, the story of the two blind men does not indicate that anyone was telling them *to be quiet.* That story says the two blind men followed Jesus and later encountered him in a home. Their persistence caused them to follow Him despite the difficulties in traveling that blindness would cause. Here in this story, Bartimaeus continues to *cry out all the more* when the crowd tries to silence him. Bartimaeus could have listened to the discouragement of the crowd and Christ would have passed him by. He could have erroneously *reasoned* that his blindness must be God's will. In contrast, Bartimaeus would not be denied his blessing. His persistence in *crying out* to Christ was rewarded because Christ stopped and took notice of him. Here is the second part of the story of Bartimaeus:

> *And Jesus stopped and said, "Call him here." And they called the blind man, saying to him, "Take courage, arise! He is calling for you." And casting aside his cloak, he jumped up, and came to Jesus. And answering him, Jesus said, "What do you want Me to do for you?" And the blind man said to Him," Rabboni, I want to regain my sight! " And Jesus*

said to him, "Go your way; your faith has made you well." And immediately he regained his sight and began following Him on the road. Mark 10:49-52

The second part of this account of healing reveals some important principles of receiving healing.

- *And Jesus stopped and said, "Call him here." And they called the blind man, saying to him, "Take courage, arise! He is calling for you." And casting aside his cloak, he jumped up, and came to Jesus.*

The same crowd that had moments before discouraged Bartimaeus, now tells him that Jesus is calling him. Everything about the description of this man's reaction reveals faith. He *cast aside his cloak.* This action reveals Bartimaeus' intense focus on the matter at hand. Nothing and no one would hinder his coming to Christ, his Healer. Bartimaeus was not playing it safe, cautious or conservative. He was radically committed to his healing. Bartimaeus believed that his blindness would be healed and that he would be able to find his cloak later. Bartimaeus does not just stand up after casting his cloak aside, he *jumps up* and comes to Jesus. Bartimaeus knew what he wanted and expressed no doubts about the will of God in his healing.

- *And the blind man said to Him," Rabboni, I want to regain my sight! " And Jesus said to him, "Go your way; your faith has made you well." And immediately he regained his sight and began following Him on the road.*

Performing Miracles and Healing

Christ does not question this man as He did the two blind men. It appears that Christ does not even have a chance to do so. Bartimaeus made his request known without any ambivalence, hesitation or doubt. Bartimaeus did not question the will of God on the matter nor did Christ. Bartimaeus simply said that he *wanted to regain his sight*. Without any hesitation or prayer, Christ tells Bartimaeus in response that *your faith has made you well*. Immediately, Bartimaeus was able to see and then followed Christ.

The elements of this story strongly contradict the idea that the Father's will is mysterious in miracles and healing. The elements in this story challenge the idea that healing is a sovereign and unpredictable act of God where God chooses one to heal and one to remain sick. In fact, Bartimaeus would not have been healed if he had believed this. Bartimaeus believed it was God's will for him to be whole and he acted on it.

In his persistence, Bartimaeus demonstrated his determined focus and strong commitment that he grasped the concept that healing is *not automatically received* but requires our participation. Doctrine that over-emphasizes the sovereignty of God as the giver and under-emphasizes the responsibility of humanity as the receiver produces passivity in people. Passive attitudes are seldom rewarded in Scripture. Indeed, much encouragement is found throughout the Bible to actively seek God for that which He alone can provide. Bartimaeus believed that he should be healed and would not be discouraged until he had received what he needed from Christ. His faith was rewarded in that he received his sight. Any person actively seeking God for healing will find that the Holy Spirit progressively builds up their faith to know that Christ is their Healer. The Spirit will then provide a circumstance where that person will encounter Christ as Healer and receive their healing.

Bethsaida's Blind Man

This story is found only in the Gospel of Mark. It has some unusual aspects. It allows for the possibility that a partial healing might be received at first.

> *And they came to Bethsaida. And they brought a blind man to Him, and entreated Him to touch him. And taking the blind man by the hand, He brought him out of the village; and after spitting on his eyes, and laying His hands upon him, He asked him, "Do you see anything?" And he looked up and said, "I see men, for I am seeing them like trees, walking about." Then again He laid His hands upon his eyes; and he looked intently and was restored, and began to see everything clearly. And He sent him to his home, saying, "Do not even enter the village."*
> *Mark 8:22-26*

There are encouraging truths about healing in this passage that are almost always apparent in New Testament teaching on this subject.

- *And they came to Bethsaida. And they brought a blind man to Him, and entreated Him to touch him.*

Performing Miracles and Healing

As in many previous situations, Christ's reputation as a Healer caused others to bring the sick, the injured, the blind and the lame to Him. There was faith that Christ could and would help this blind man by a simple touch.

- _And taking the blind man by the hand, He brought him out of the village..._

Exactly _why_ Christ took this man out of the village of Bethsaida is not entirely evident here. The passage does not comment on it. On the other hand, Christ said some very pointed and negative things about Bethsaida. He compared it and several other cities with Tyre and Sidon on the day of judgement. These two sinful Old Testament cities experienced God's judgement by their destruction. Christ said this about Bethsaida:

> _Then He began to reproach the cities in which most of His miracles were done, because they did not repent. "Woe to you, Chorazin! Woe to you, Bethsaida! For if the miracles had occurred in Tyre and Sidon which occurred in you, they would have repented long ago in sackcloth and ashes._
> _Mark 11:20-21_

Christ was obviously disappointed in the response of Bethsaida to the miracles in His ministry. The two miracles of the feeding of the four and five thousand happened near Bethsaida. Additionally, various texts imply that thousands of people were healed in this region.

Christ Heals the Blind

The eyewitnesses in Bethsaida and Chorazin should have *repented* when they saw Christ's wonderful miraculous works. Bethsaida had not responded to Christ properly. It is possible to speculate on why Christ took this blind man outside Bethsaida to heal him. Perhaps, despite Christ's miracles in the village of Bethsaida, there was serious religious opposition to Him. Perhaps Christ needed to take the blind man out of this city because unbelieving opposition had arisen. Perhaps, for the conditions to be right for the blind man to receive this miracle, this blind man needed to be away from those who would criticize the healing. Perhaps, the blind man's faith was weak and fragile. In any case, Christ created new conditions for the blind man before He ministered to him.

- *and after spitting on his eyes, and laying His hands upon him, He asked him, "Do you see anything?"*

This is the only place recorded in the Gospels where Christ uses the particular methodology of directly spitting on a man. Occasionally, the Gospel writers recorded an unusual methodology in healing. The only similar event in Christ's recorded ministry is the healing event where Christ spit on the ground and made clay and applied the clay to the eyes of a man born blind. That event of healing, recorded in John's Gospel, will be reviewed at the end of this chapter.

The Holy Spirit occasionally reveals an unusual methodology that must be obeyed in order for the healing to occur. No one should ever think that such unusual methodologies are the norm. They are not. In most cases, healing will occur without a word of knowledge being involved or an unusual method. In this story, Christ also uses a normal method: the laying on of hands.

- *...and laying His hands upon him...*

As with many other accounts of the ministry of Christ, laying on of hands is revealed as Christ's ongoing method of choice in healing ministry. He needed no specific guidance to do this healing. Christ *already* knew the will of the Father in matters of healing. The Father wants people well. However, Christ maintained *openness* to specific guidance from the Holy Spirit of *how* to heal someone.

- *...He asked him, "Do you see anything?"*

This question reveals a great deal. It reveals that Christ did not know exactly *what* the man would experience. If there is any mystery in healing and miracles, it lies in this area. While there is no mystery in the Father's will, *what* a believing person experiences may be a surprise. They may feel divine heat. They may feel the Holy Spirit's power in the form of living electricity. They may feel a demon leave. They may feel nothing at all but their pain is gone. They may receive a partial healing that will strongly encourage them to seek Christ for the completion of their healing.

Christ understood that this healing was not based on what He believed but rather was based upon what the man believed. The circumstances of this healing may reveal the fragility of the faith of this particular blind man. Christ may have understood that He must work with this man through his healing in order for him to receive. This might have been the reason that Christ took him out of Bethsaida. Christ might have known that this man would be overly sensitive to false *accusation* directed at either Christ or him personally. In any case, Christ asks the question and gets this answer from the man.

- *And he looked up and said, "I see men, for I am seeing them like trees, walking about."*

The blind man received a partial healing. He was aware that he was seeing the people around him and their movements, but they appeared as *trees* to him. In other words, he could not yet see detail and depth. Instantaneous healing is not the only expression of Christ's healing ministry. Where a partial healing is received, strong faith for finishing the healing ought to result. This kind of sanctified logic ought to motivate the believer: *If the Father was willing to do this much, He is willing to finish the healing. If I was able to receive partially, then I am able to receive the rest of my healing even if I must receive it in stages as my faith grows.*

After getting the man's response, Christ *again* placed His hands upon the man's eyes.

- *Then again He laid His hands upon his eyes...*

Christ did not settle for a partial healing. Christ knew that the Father's will for this man was complete wholeness *despite* how slowly the man received healing. This is why Christ did *not* hesitate at all to lay his hands again on the man. For someone to have an *authentic* ministry that models itself on Christ's example, allowance must be made for an occasional situation like this. In a very few cases, counseling a person through their healing may be the only way to get them healed. The results of Christ laying His hands again on this man are revealing.

- *and he looked intently and was restored, and began to see everything clearly.*

The Father's will was revealed in the man getting his complete sight. The time interval between his partial healing and his complete healing seems short but is clearly long enough for the conversation to take place and for the man to evaluate just how much he was seeing.

It seems wise to allow for partial healings as an encouragement to believe for complete healings. Faith may not be great enough initially to receive a complete healing but enough to receive something from God. In other words, if a partial healing is received, then the person receiving should believe with greater conviction that the Father desires them to receive complete healing. Anyone wishing to accomplish healing like the Savior must be willing to do it like He did. Christ finishes His ministry to this man by some specific instruction.

- *And He sent him to his home, saying, "Do not even enter the village."*

Christ Heals the Blind

This man was not from Bethsaida. His home was elsewhere. Christ obviously did not want this man to enter Bethsaida for unexplained reasons that were speculated upon above.

The Man Born Blind

This story, found in John's Gospel, is the only specifically mentioned case of a birth defect being healed. There were probably many others, but this is the only place where the writer has explicitly declared that particular information. This story is very important since Christ declared the purpose of God for the birth defect. The issue of who should be blamed for birth defects also appears in the story. This story is very long and fills a complete chapter in John's Gospel. The last half of the story tells what happened to the man after he was healed. While this is interesting information, we will not review the last half of the story. Here is the first half of the story which describes the man's healing:

And as He (Christ) passed by (the Temple), He saw a man blind from birth. And His disciples asked Him, saying, "Rabbi, who sinned, this man or his parents, that he should be born blind?" Jesus answered, "It was neither that this man sinned, nor his parents; but it was in order that the works of God might be displayed in him. We must work the works of Him who sent Me, as long as it is day; night is coming, when no man can work. While I am in the world, I am the light of the world." When He had said this, He spat on the ground, and made clay of the spittle, and applied the clay to his eyes, and said to him, "Go, wash in the pool of Siloam" (which is translated, Sent). And so he went away and washed, and came back seeing. John 9:1-7

This passage has interesting and important theological implications. In it, Christ offers information in the realm of the purpose of God for birth defects that no other passage offers.

- *And as He (Christ) passed by (the Temple), He saw a man blind from birth.*

Christ left the Temple area after a sharp verbal exchange with the hostile Jewish leaders. This information is found in Chapter 8 of John's Gospel. After leaving Christ saw this blind man, probably among the beggars around the Temple area. The text says that Christ *saw* this man. However, since the disciples asked Him about this particular man, Christ apparently stopped and looked directly at the man and that behavior apparently spurred this question from His disciples.

- *And His disciples asked Him, saying, "Rabbi, who sinned, this man or his parents, that he should be born blind?"*

What an important question! The disciples want to know *who or what* is to *blame* for this man's birth defect. They make the assumption that someone's sin must be the cause. They want to know if the man is to blame because of his sin or his parent's sins. Of course, the logic of the blind man's sins being the cause of his blindness is weak even before Christ's answer. Since the man was born blind, this would have God disciplining the man *before* he had an opportunity to sin. The logic of God punishing a child for the parent's sin is not much better. However, Scripture does validate that a parent's sins can cause difficulties in the lives of their children, so this could be a possibility. It is easy to see experientially that the sins of parents do often affect their children negatively. Christ's answer, however, dismisses that possibility in this case.

- *Jesus answered, "It was neither that this man sinned, nor his parents...*

Christ makes it clear that *sin* was *not* the direct cause of this birth defect. This is important. It helps believers avoid the *blame game*. The *blame game* is the sinful tendency of humanity to want to fix the blame for difficulties upon someone. The *blame game* is normally very counterproductive to the healing and deliverance of people. Christ, with very few exceptions, does not address the relationship of sin with healing. Normally, Christ healed people without saying a word about their sins or what caused the sickness and without fixing blame. However, in His public preaching of the Kingdom of God, repentance was an important part. In other words, Christ's public ministry called people to repentance, but in His ongoing ministry to individuals, He seldom said anything about their need to repent. Christ just showed them the mercy of the Father and healed them.

Three kinds of persons are often blamed for sickness or disability. First, the actual victims of the condition are blamed. While there are times when someone brings a condition upon himself or herself, Christ seldom addresses the source of the condition beyond telling the person to *sin no more*. This encouragement not to sin again took place *after* the person was healed. In many cases, the behavior of a person has nothing to do with their condition, as in this story. Secondly, the parents or spouses are blamed. While relatives might have had some responsibility, normally this is not the case either. Christ does not blame anyone for sickness. He simply heals the sick despite the source of their problems. Thirdly, blame is *most often* fixed on God. This is often very subtle and cloaked by religiosity. This hidden blame is theologically explained, and sickness and debilitating conditions are transformed into a mysterious blessing from the Father.

It is difficult for someone who loses a child to sickness, or suffers a debilitating and painful condition, to continue to maintain faith in a God that they believe is responsible for their suffering and untimely loss. Sometimes the responsibility for the loss is given to God by two logical arguments. First, they believe that God must have had a mysterious planned purpose for the suffering or the untimely death. This logic seems to overlook that Scripture often reveals that the work of demons is directly responsible for some sickness and disability. Secondly, since God did not apparently come to the suffering person's aid, then they believe that it must not be His will to heal. This logic seems to forget that there are specific conditions to be met in receiving healing.

Christ Heals the Blind

Doubts about God's goodness are often hidden in the sincere people wounded by such circumstances. These good people will normally maintain that they believe that God is good and have found solace in God's mercy and grace. However, these same people will often have problems thereafter in finding faith for healing and other personal matters. The truth is that the Father is not to blame for their pain. He would have it otherwise. He sent Christ to bear their sins, sicknesses and pain. Therefore, it is much better not to fix the blame on anyone but rather to encourage those who experience loss to continue to look to a faithful and gracious Father.

In this situation, Christ refuses to fix the blame on anyone. He explains the purpose of God for this man's condition very differently. Christ answers the question of who is to blame differently than most theological expressions do today.

- *...but it was in order that the works of God might be displayed in him.*

Christ reveals that this man had this condition simply because the Father wanted to *display* publicly that He had healed him. His condition of blindness did not bring God any glory. As long as the man was blind, he simply was one of many undistinguished beggars. His healing glorified the Father not his disability.

This man's healing caused him to have an extraordinary testimony. This man became a powerful witness of God's power through Jesus Christ. Everyone in this locality knew that this man had been born blind. The facts of his healing should have been indisputable. However, as the last half of the chapter relates, this man's public healing caused a great stir, controversy and opposition among the religious leaders. There were many people healed in Jerusalem but this man's testimony was indisputable. The unbelieving religious opposition to Christ found great difficulty explaining it away.

The longer that an individual has been suffering and the more serious their illness or condition, the greater glory will God receive when they are healed. How strong their testimony will be when they are healed! However, no one should ever believe that they should wait to be healed to bring God additional glory. The price has *already* been paid at the cross. Today is the day of salvation. Today is the day of healing. Christ healed people *immediately* wherever and whenever He encountered them. He did not send people away to return later to increase the glory[3].

This healing should encourage anyone suffering from a birth defect or any long-term illness. Many of the healings recorded in the Gospels were people with serious long-term conditions. For instance, Christ healed the woman who had a twelve-year hemorrhage and the woman who had been afflicted by a demon for eighteen years[4]. The Gospel writers purposely recorded these healings with the details of *how long* these people were ill. Obviously,

---

[3] The resurrection of Lazarus is the only possible exception. Christ purposely waited until Lazarus had been dead four days before He came to Bethsaida to resurrect Him. However, Lazarus would have been already dead even if He had arrived as soon as possible. We will review this story later in this text.

[4] These two stories are found in Luke 8:43-48 and Luke 13:10-17

the length of time that a person has a particular condition *in no way reveals* that the condition is will of the Father. When these people first encountered Christ the Healer, they were immediately made well. The work that Christ received from the Father was to reveal the Father's will and works. The Father wanted those people with long-term illnesses and conditions well from the beginning.

- *We must work the works of Him who sent Me...*

Christ worked the works of the Father who sent Him. However, what Christ says above includes His disciples. Instead of saying *I,* Christ says *we.* Christ had just healed the man born blind and then tells His disciples that *we* must *work the works* of the Father. This is clear encouragement for them to do the same kinds of miraculous works.

Additionally, the work of the Father was healing this man. Nothing in this passage indicates that the work of the Father was happening *before* this man's healing. There is nothing in this passage that reveals that some mysterious work of the Father was happening in this man by virtue of his condition of blindness. However, the only work of the Father that is revealed in this passage is this man's healing.

Christ says that, *"We must work the works of the Father."* This phrase reveals the human-Divine relationship in healing and miracle ministry. While these are the Father's works, *we* must work them. While God does heal without using a human vessel, that is not His preferred way. In the Church age, the Father most often reveals Christ the Healer through human vessels. In fact, in the New Testament, it is unusual for someone to be healed without God somehow using a human instrument in the process of healing. While believers are powerless to help on our own, the Father empowers them in Christ to end suffering by healing and delivering.

- *...as long as it is day; night is coming, when no man can work.*

Believers are to *work the works* of the Father while they have opportunity. Christ reveals that opportunity will not be present at all times in the future. For Himself, the night was coming and His opportunities to *work the works* of the Father were at an end. If opportunity still exists, then the *day* is present and believers should be *working the works* of the Father.

- *While I am in the world, I am the light of the world.*

Christ knew that His time for ministry was limited and His time within the world was ending. While in the world, Christ was the light of the world. However, He knew that the time was approaching when *His disciples* would be *the light of the world*[5] revealing Him by reproducing His ministry.

- *When He had said this, He spat on the ground, and made clay of the spittle, and applied the clay to his eyes...*

---

[5] *"You are the light of the world..."* Matthew 5:14a

Christ Heals the Blind

This was the second time that Christ used spittle in some way to heal. In this case, a practical concern may have been present. The blind man would not have been able to see Christ making the clay. The blind man simply would have felt something cool being applied to his eyes. The clay would have provided a temporary feeling to the man's eyes even after it dried that might have helped him believe.

- *and said to him, "Go, wash in the pool of Siloam" (which is translated, Sent). And so he went away and washed, and came back seeing.*

The pool of Siloam had a reputation as being a place of healing among the Jews. Beyond the clay on the man's eyes, Christ might have been using something practical to aid the man's faith. Christ chose a pool that was well known as a place of healing to possibly help this man's faith. Christ sent the blind man to the *healing* pool to wash the clay off. By obedience to Christ's command to wash in this pool, the man was demonstrating his faith. Obviously, all movement to a blind person is difficult. Movement to a place that the blind man ordinarily did not go would be much more difficult. However, obedience to Christ's command, difficult as it may be, demonstrated that the blind man believed he would be healed. Otherwise, he would have not made the effort to go there, since he would realize that he would also have to make the trip back. Whether or not he was assisted is not revealed in the passage. Nevertheless, the man's obedient faith was rewarded. He was blind no longer.

Performing Miracles and Healing

One of the reasons that this chapter comes early in the specific events of Christ's healing is that some see healing the blind at the top of the list of difficult healings. This belief is unfortunate since it appears that blindness was no more difficult for Christ than any other kind of healing. Sanctified logic should be applied here. Believers have no power in themselves, without Christ, to heal anyone of anything. However, Christ within them can do all things well. Believers can neither fail nor succeed in healing. Christ alone heals the sick. If healing the blind was not hard for Christ then, it is not hard for Him now. _One thing is no harder than another_. One healing is no more difficult than another. If Christ will heal a cold through a believer, then blindness is no harder for Him. Believers must understand that Christ lives within them, and that He is capable of doing great miracles despite their insecurities and feelings of inadequacy. In fact, when we realize the inability and inadequacy of our flesh, and His great ability working through us, this brings glory to God. The Holy Spirit releases power to do the works of the Father to anyone who knows by faith that Christ is always capable and willing to do mighty things through flawed human vessels.

~7~

Christ Heals Infections & Fevers

John the Baptist sent some of his disciples to Christ to ask Him if He was the predicted Messiah. Christ identified His ministry to John the Baptist by describing it in some detail. Here is what Christ said about His own ministry to John's disciples:

> ...*Go and report to John what you hear and see: the BLIND RECEIVE SIGHT and the lame walk, the lepers are cleansed and the deaf hear, and the dead are raised up, and the POOR HAVE THE GOSPEL PREACHED TO THEM.* Matthew 11:4-5

One of the special things that is identified in Christ's ministry is that the *lepers are cleansed*. Christ also commanded the Twelve, and us by implication, to do the same things.

Heal the sick, raise the dead, cleanse the lepers, cast out demons; freely you received, freely give. Matthew 10:8

Since Christ has identified this specific miraculous work, the specific accounts of this type of healing are worth considering first in this chapter.

The Cleansing of the Ten Lepers

This story, found in the Gospel of Luke, Chapter 17, teaches a great deal about the will of the Father and the place of faith in healing.

> *And as He entered a certain village, ten leprous men who stood at a distance met Him; and they raised their voices, saying, "Jesus, Master, have mercy on us!" And when He saw them, He said to them, "Go and show yourselves to the priests." And it came about that as they were going, they were cleansed. Now one of them, when he saw that he had been healed, turned back, glorifying God with a loud voice, and he fell on his face at His feet, giving thanks to Him. And he was a Samaritan. And Jesus answered and said, "Were there not ten cleansed? But the nine-- where are they? Was no one found who turned back to give glory to God, except this foreigner?" And He said to him, "Rise, and go your way; your faith has made you well." Luke 17:12-19*

This passage has many familiar elements and a few new and interesting things as well:

Christ Heals Infections and Fevers

- *And as He entered a certain village, ten leprous men who stood at a distance met Him; and they raised their voices, saying, "Jesus, Master, have mercy on us!"*

These ten men *stood at a distance* from Christ. People with leprosy were social outcasts and uninfected people scattered in fear when they were near. Lepers were believed to be under the judgement of God for their sins, and therefore, they were due no mercy. They were continually rejected by the people around them, which added to the problems of a progressively horrible disease. Additionally, the Law of Moses forbade those who were infected to live with healthy people. The Law imposed a wise quarantine thousands of years before anything was known of germs or how infectious illness spreads. These lepers had to live *outside the camp* of the healthy. This meant that they seldom had adequate shelter, food or clothing.

The progression of this disease leaves the infected without feeling in their hands and feet. They have open sores on the hands and feet because they continually injure themselves due to the lack of feeling. Eventually, they may lose their fingers, toes and portions of their faces such as their noses or ears.

Leprosy is contagious, although not extremely so. It can be spread by physical contact with the leprous person, particularly if the contact is ongoing. Because the disease produces insensitivity in the hands and feet, and a serious dryness and cracking of the skin, serious injuries and subsequent infections are often a side-effect of the disease.

Amputations and serious scarring are common among those who are untreated. Disfigurement of leprous persons creates fear in the uninfected. This fear element is similar to the fears of modern plague of AIDS. In fact, AIDS might be called "the modern leprosy".

Both diseases, AIDS and leprosy, have an element of shame that society attaches to them. In the ancient world, leprosy was seen as a judgement from God. Indeed, there were examples of God judging sin with leprosy, sometimes temporarily, sometimes not, in the Old Testament. Today, many think that AIDS is a judgement from God. Many think that those infected with AIDS somehow deserve the disease because they may have acted irresponsibly in illegal intravenous drug use or a sexual matter. Of course, in the case of leprosy or AIDS, innocents sometimes become infected as well. In any case, whether responsible for their illness or not, Christ deals with them all the same.

- *And* when He saw them, He said to *them, "Go and show yourselves to the priests."*

Christ responded in a positive manner to the ten lepers. By telling them to g*o and show yourselves to the priests*, Christ was telling them that they were to respond to what the Law of Moses said to do in order to be received back into society. The Law of Moses had a specific process whereby the priest determined if someone who had a contagious disease had become well. Christ was telling them to go through this process of being declared healed. If the lepers had not believed that they were healed, they would not have left the presence of Christ. They understood what going to the priest meant. Perhaps some of them had prayed and dreamt of the day when they might go to a priest to be declared well.

- *And it came about that as they were going, they were cleansed.*

Their faith in Christ resulted in obedience to His direction. Their expression of faith resulted in their healing. This would have been an ideal opportunity for the Holy Spirit to demonstrate that the Father's will is different for different people. Instead, all ten lepers were healed without any consideration of whether or not their serious illnesses, pain and deformity might have been doing some kind of unspecified mysterious good in their lives.

The New Testament has a specific word connected to the healing of leprosy. These ten men were *cleansed* from leprosy. *Cleansing* is a translation of a form of the Greek word *katharizo*. This word means *to purify, to purge, to make spotless and clean[1]*.

This Greek word is used in the New Testament in reference to the removal of physical stains and dirt from utensils. The Old Testament included ceremonial washing of utensils to make them *clean*. This Greek word is also used in reference to the removal of the defilement of sin, corrupt desire, and guilt. In many places in the Gospels, this Greek word is used in reference to the healing of the infectious disease leprosy.

---

[1] Vines, pg. 186-187

Performing Miracles and Healing

Healing of leprosy was *to purify, to purge, to make the leprous person spotless and clean* in a *physical* but also in a *moral* sense. Healing of leprosy was seen as forgiveness and the removal of judgement on the person. If the formerly leprous person was now healed, the priest was to declare them *cleansed* and then they were able to return to their families and Hebrew society.

- *Now one of them, when he saw that he had been healed, turned back, glorifying God with a loud voice, and he fell on his face at His feet, giving thanks to Him. And he was a Samaritan.*

One of the ten that was healed had a different reaction than the other nine. The passage tells us of four actions on his part in response to being healed. Two were physical actions with his body: He *turned back* and *fell on his face.* Two were actions with his voice: He *glorified God with a loud voice* and *gave thanks* to Christ. His physical reactions reflected great humility and the actions with his voice reflect *praise and thanksgiving.* Luke tells us that this man was a Samaritan rather than a Jew. Christ's reaction to this man reveals that the Samaritan had the proper reaction to the situation.

- *And Jesus answered and said, "Were there not ten cleansed? But the nine-- where are they? Was no one found who turned back to give glory to God, except this foreigner?"*

It was necessary to *turn back* in order to *give glory to God.* This shows that this man had made the connection between Christ and the Father. This man saw the Father at work in Christ and knew that he must *return* to Christ in order to *give glory to God*. The passage does not say why the other nine did not turn back. It is clear that they did not see the Father in Christ or they would have reacted in the same manner. Perhaps they were afraid not to do exactly what Christ had said. Perhaps they thought of God as a heavy-handed taskmaster that would take back their healing if they failed to mechanically execute every detail of Christ's words. Of course, it is not logical to believe that a God who heals would be less gracious to someone who took time to be thankful. Perhaps, they were not as thankful as the Samaritan and were focused upon returning to their old lives. In any case, Christ's surprised reaction to the nine not returning tells us that they obviously failed to react properly. Apparently, there is always time to praise and be thankful in God's plan. Christ's surprise also again reveals that He did not know everything in advance.

- *And He said to him, "Rise, and go your way; your faith has made you well."*

Christ tells this man the same truth that He had repeatedly told others in similar situations. The Samaritan's *faith has made him well*. This was true of the other nine as well but they didn't get to hear it from Christ. In other situations, *healing* resulted from the seeking Christ in faith. In this case, a particular kind of healing, a *cleansing*, has occurred as a result of the Samaritan's faith in Christ.

There are several other important things to be learned through the cleansing of the ten lepers. First of all, even though nine of the lepers had a less than proper response to the healing, they were still healed. For those who think that God requires some sort of perfection of faith and attitudes before healing is received, this situation reveals something different. God knew that nine of these men would not respond entirely properly but that did not limit His grace to them. What we see here is the graciousness and mercy of God being revealed. Secondly, this situation of ten men being healed all at once would have been a perfect place for God to reveal that His will in healing might be different for different people. God could have shown distinctions between these men by healing only a few of them. Instead, Christ heals all ten leprous men without distinction or qualification beyond the faith that was required by their coming to Christ.

Another Specific Cleansing of A Leper

There is a second detailed account of the healing of leprosy. This account is found in Matthew Chapter 8. There is another account of the same event found in Mark 1:40-44. Instead of ten men being cleansed from leprosy, it reveals Christ's interaction with a single unnamed leper. This man could be Simon the Leper who is mentioned in Matthew 26:6 and Mark 14:3.

> *And when He had come down from the mountain, great multitudes followed Him. And behold, a leper came to Him, and bowed down to Him, saying, "Lord, if You are willing, You can make me clean." And He stretched out His hand and touched him, saying, "I am willing; be cleansed." And immediately his leprosy was cleansed. And Jesus*

said to him, "See that you tell no one; but go, show yourself to the priest, and present the offering that Moses commanded, for a testimony to them." Matthew 8:1-4

Various truths reveal themselves in this passage. Many are familiar and help us to review some common truths revealed repeatedly in Christ's ministry.

- *And when He had come down from the mountain, great multitudes followed Him. And behold, a leper came to Him, and bowed down to Him...*

Christ had just finished the discourse that has been traditionally called the Sermon on the Mount. This is the *mountain* referred to in the passage. Amidst the great multitude following him, a leper came and humbled himself before Christ by bowing.

- *... saying, "Lord, if You are willing, You can make me clean."*

The leper first addresses Christ as *Lord*. This is the from the Greek word *kurios*. This term simply means *one who has authority*. It is sometimes translated *master* and even as *owner*. This is often confused with the word *LORD* that has a different meaning. *LORD*, written with all capital letters, is a word that translators substitute for a word associated with a particular name for God.

The apostle Paul writes in his letter to the Philippians that everyone will eventually say... *Jesus*

Christ is Lord. It is another way of saying that *Jesus the Messiah is the King.* In this passage, Paul uses the same Greek word as the leper above. In other words, the leper was acknowledging the authority of Christ and perhaps His power to heal him.

The leper makes a statement to Christ that has an implicit question in it. The leper knows that Christ has the power to heal him. What the leper is *not entirely sure* about is whether it is *the will of God* for Christ to heal him. Many people today come to the same emotional and spiritual place of this leper. They understand and believe in Christ's ability to help them. What they doubt is His willingness to help them. Much modern theology has taught these theological doubts rather than Christ's reactions to people in Scripture. This is the only place in the New Testament where the question of Christ's *willingness to heal* is addressed in *a direct way.* Christ's reaction to this man ought to instruct believers about what the Father's will is in such matters.

- *And He stretched out His hand and touched him, saying, "I am willing; be cleansed." And immediately his leprosy was cleansed.*

Christ does not hesitate. Christ does not pray to the Father to understand His will in this specific circumstance. Christ *already knows* the will of the Father in these matters. The Father's will is to heal, make whole, set free and in this particular case to cleanse. He immediately touches the leper and states that, *"I am willing."*

Christ Heals Infections and Fevers

Christ does not give the leper a theological dissertation about the will of the Father and healing. His verbal expression comes from simple compassion for this suffering man that results in his healing. In fact, the parallel account of this healing in Mark's Gospel offers this small but revealing addition to the account.

And moved with compassion, He stretched out His hand, and touched him, and said to him, "I am willing; be cleansed." Mark 1:41

Much modern theology produces complex emotional and theological reactions to sick or injured people that limit compassion and faith for healing. This theology produces fears that the person will be spiritually injured by possible failure in believing God for healing. Those embracing this complex theology somehow think that remaining sick or injured would be better.

Normally, there is some illogical behavior found with this complex theology. The same afflicted people would seek medical help from a doctor. Yet, they apply these odd ideas to their relationship with God. If they actually believed that the injury, sickness or suffering was the will of God, and therefore doing some mysterious good, they would not seek a doctor. In other words, this theology produces fears that seeking God for healing will ruin some mysterious dealing from God that they are willing to ruin themselves by seeking a doctor. Christ did not have this kind of complex emotional and theological reaction to this leprous man. He simply was _moved with compassion_ and consequently _cleansed_ him from leprosy.

Christ's reaction after this man was cleansed is rather different than many modern expressions of ministry.

- *And Jesus said to him, "See that you tell no one; but go, show yourself to the priest, and present the offering that Moses commanded, for a testimony to them."*

Christ tells them to *tell no one*. Christ did not want to advertise Himself. Perhaps Christ's concern was for the cleansed leper and not for His own reputation. Christ then tells the cleansed leper to go through the process that the Law of Moses reveals in order that a testimony might be given to those who are priests. This would be similar to someone who had been healed going back to the doctor to insure that their healing is complete as a testimony to the medical profession. The motive of their returning to the doctor would not be doubt or fear that they had not be healed, but a desire for Christ to be glorified as Healer to the medical community.

Royal Official's Son Sick with Fever

The third account of a healing from what appears to have been an infection of some sort is found in the Gospel of John. Here is the first half of the story:

He came therefore again to Cana of Galilee where He had made the water wine. And there was a certain royal official, whose son was sick at Capernaum. When he heard that Jesus had come out of Judea into Galilee, he went to Him, and was requesting Him to come down and heal his son; for he was at the point of death. Jesus therefore said to him, "Unless you people see signs and wonders, you simply will not believe." John 4:46-48

Christ returned to Cana in Galilee from the region of Judea. Apparently, Christ was the *talk of the town* because a royal official living in another town in the region heard that Christ had returned. This royal official may have been a relative of King Herod or one of his sons. This group of people was called the *Herodians* and generally opposed Christ along with the religious Pharisees. However, the Herodians were more political than religious and worked with the Romans to control the Jewish people.

- *He (Christ) came therefore again to Cana of Galilee where He had made the water wine. And there was a certain royal official, whose son was sick at Capernaum. When he heard that Jesus had come out of Judea into Galilee, he went to Him, and was requesting Him to come down and heal his son; for he was at the point of death.*

This royal official knew that Christ had been healing people and his son's nearness to death made him seek out Christ. He desperately wanted Christ to come with him to *Capernaum* to heal his son. Christ's response is different than His response to parents of sick children in other places. Christ's response shows that He perceived a problem in the man's request. These words and tone seems very much like a correction of the royal official's lack of faith:

- _Jesus therefore said to him, "Unless you people see signs and wonders, you simply will not believe."_

Christ reproves an unspecified _you people_ for a _failure to believe_. Christ is obviously including the royal official in His statement. Christ seems to be reproving the _Herodians_ as a group of people for not believing without seeing signs and wonders. Obviously, Christ is not being critical of signs and wonders in His own ministry. He is correcting this man's, and his particular class of people's, failure to believe without seeing signs and wonders. The royal official apparently received the correction properly. Here is the rest of the story:

> _The royal official said to Him, "Sir, come down before my child dies." Jesus said to him, "Go your way; your son lives." The man believed the word that Jesus spoke to him, and he started off. And as he was now going down, his slaves met him, saying that his son was living. So he inquired of them the hour when he began to get better. They said therefore to him, "Yesterday at the seventh hour the fever left him." So the father knew that it was at that hour in which Jesus said to him, "Your son lives"; and he himself believed, and his whole household. This is again a second sign that Jesus performed, when He had come out of Judea into Galilee._
> _John 4:49-54_

This royal official apparently humbled himself to receive Christ's correction about him not believing. The official continued to seek Christ after the reproof rather than being insulted.

- *The royal official said to Him, "Sir, come down before my child dies."*

The royal official still wanted Christ to come with him to heal his child. This is perhaps where Christ had perceived a problem with the man's faith. The royal official was in *desperation* wanting to *see* Christ heal his son. However, desperation is *not* faith. Faith is *not* based on *seeing*. Faith is the evidence of things *not yet seen*. However, something seems to be different after this man received Christ's correction. Perhaps this man had begun to believe without seeing.

- *Jesus said to him, "Go your way; your son lives." The man believed the word that Jesus spoke to him, and he started off.*

It appears that the moment that the man started believing, an unusual miracle resulted. Christ then received revelation, a word of knowledge, that the dying son had been healed and stated that fact to the royal official. In this case, it seems that Christ was reporting that the healing had *already been done.*[2] The royal official then *believed* Christ's word without actually seeing his son's healing.

---

[2] There is another way to look at this healing which is also possible. Perhaps the man first believed when he heard Christ pronounce that his son was healed. However, the author thinks the language of the passage lends itself best to the interpretation above and this interpretation is theologically consistent with other passages. However, the other interpretation is not bad

- *And as he was now going down, his slaves met him, saying that his son was living. So he inquired of them the hour when he began to get better. They said therefore to him, "Yesterday at the seventh hour the fever left him." So the father knew that it was at that hour in which Jesus said to him, "Your son lives..."*

The synagogue official inquired as to what time his son began to get well. He discovered that his son was healed at precisely the time when he had the discussion with Christ. Precise timing is often the way that the Father demonstrates that healing or some other intervention has come divinely rather than naturally.

The account above also indicates that the son's nearness to death was a result of a *fever.* What exactly caused this *fever* is unknown. It could have been an infection or some other malady. The Greek word that is translated *fever* in this passage is *puretos,* which comes from the Greek word *pur* that means *fire.* What is clear is that this child was *burning with fever* and not expected to live. Because of the father's faith in Christ as Healer a remarkable miracle happened, the fever left at the precise time that Christ told the father that the child was well at some distance away.

- *and he himself believed, and his whole household.*

This is the third time where *believing* is mentioned in this account. The first time was Christ correcting the

---

either. Both interpretations emphasize faith and persistence in receiving healing.

royal official. The second time was after Christ pronounced that the child was healed. The third time is in the statement above. Each time during this situation, the royal official's *faith* in Christ grew stronger and his testimony of his son's healing caused his whole household to believe in Christ.

- *This is again a second sign that Jesus performed, when He had come out of Judea into Galilee.*

The apostle John refers to this healing as *a second sign*. The first sign was Christ turning the water into wine at the wedding in Cana. John also says that Jesus *performed* these *signs*. This implies that Christ had some control of healing and miracles.

The Healing of Peter's Mother-in-law

Christ's ministry extended to the families of his disciples. Early in his ministry, just after casting out a demon out of a man in the synagogue at Capernaum, these events occurred:

And He (Christ) arose and left the synagogue, and entered Simon's home. Now Simon's mother-in-law was suffering from a high fever; and they made request of Him on her behalf. And standing over her, He rebuked the fever, and it left her; and she immediately arose and waited on them.
Luke 4:38-39

Performing Miracles and Healing

Luke gives us specific details in his precise wording in this short passage that illuminate what Christ did in this situation.

- _And He (Christ) arose and left the synagogue, and entered Simon's home. Now Simon's mother-in-law was suffering from a high fever;_

The _Simon_ that this passage is addressing is _Simon Peter_, one of Christ's twelve disciples. The passage lets us know that Peter was married by the fact that he had a mother-in-law who was ill. She was _suffering from a high fever_. The same Greek word for _fever_ is used here as in the story of the royal official's son, except for a small modifier. Luke has added the Greek word _megas_ to _puretos_ that means _great_ or _high_. Luke, the physician, is using a First Century medical classification. Physicians in Luke's day classified fevers into _great fevers_ and _little fevers_[3]. Luke is using his medical knowledge to tell his readers that Peter's mother-in-law had a _great fever_.

- _and they made request of Him on her behalf._

Who asked Christ to heal Peter's mother-in-law is not entirely clear here. However, this healing occurred _before_ Christ gathered His disciples. Peter, James, John and Matthew (Levi) were all called as disciples in the next chapter, Chapter Five, of Luke's Gospel. Since these events occurred this early in Christ's ministry, it is probable that only Peter and his family were present in this home.

---

[3] Vine's, pg. 421.

Christ Heals Infections and Fevers

- _And standing over her, He rebuked the fever, and it left her; and she immediately arose and waited on them._

She must have been lying on a mat on the floor of the house for Christ to be able to _stand over her._ People slept on the floor on mats in First Century Jewish homes. This also indicates that Christ _did not lay hands_ on her. Christ simply _spoke_ to the fever and _it left her._ The passage says that _He rebuked the fever._ Luke is extraordinarily precise in how he words these accounts. Luke repeatedly uses the same Greek word translated _rebuke_ several times in this chapter. This same Greek word is found in verses 35, 39 and 41 in this chapter. In the cases of verse 35 and 41, both times Christ is _rebuking a demon._ Sandwiched in between two accounts of Christ rebuking demons is verse 39, where Christ is _rebuking a fever._ This hints that a demon was causing the high fever in Peter's mother-in-law. Luke's use of specific language in this passage also hints that this was a demon by saying that the fever _left her_ instead of saying that she was healed. Since these are only hints, even if they are strong hints, this account is not included in the chapter that follows on sickness caused by demonic activity.

~8~

Healing and Demonic Activity

A Restored New Testament Ministry

In order to deal sufficiently with the connection between deliverance ministry and healing, the next few pages will review, in a general way, the subject of *casting out demons*. An abundance of additional material exists on this subject that cannot be specifically covered in this book. The main focus of deliverance ministry after these next few pages will be limited to these situations where a medical condition was cured after Christ cast out a demon.

Deliverance Ministry or *casting out demons* is supernatural New Testament ministry. In Churches where the authority of Jesus Christ is taught, and the fullness of the Spirit welcomed, this ministry should be seen frequently. In the past thirty years, the number of people in the United States ministering deliverance from evil spirits has grown from a few dozen to tens of thousands of believers. The Holy Spirit is cleansing the Bride of Christ from evil and making Her ready for the coming of the Bridegroom!

In churches where there is no deliverance ministry today, there are often serious problems not addressed in the lives of believers. This creates secret sins and hypocrisy in the life of the church. Eventually, because there seems to be no solution to their problems, many discouraged believers backslide under demonic pressures. However, there is a solution. The scriptural remedy must be applied to this problem.

Believers Should Cast Out Demons

Jesus commissioned His disciples by giving them authority[1] and power[2] over evil spirits. Driving out or casting out demons was to accompany their preaching, along with regular healing of the sick and other miracles.

> *"When Jesus had called the Twelve together, He gave them power and authority to drive out all demons and to cure diseases... Luke 9:1*

If healing is for today then casting out demons is for today. This authority was not granted only to the Twelve apostles. The Lord Jesus reveals the authority He has given to all believers over the power of demons.

> *The seventy-two returned with joy and said, "Lord, even the demons submit to us in your name." He replied, "I saw Satan fall like lightning from heaven.*

---

[1] Greek: *exousia*
[2] Greek: *dunamis*

I have given you authority to trample on snakes and scorpions and to overcome all the power of the enemy; nothing will harm you." Luke 10:17-19 [3]

Casting Out Demons is a Sign of Faith

Casting out demons is described as a sign that will follow believers. In other words, it is a sign of faith. Where there is true faith in Christ operating, then we would expect to see this sign. Jesus reveals this in the Gospel of Mark. Jesus commissioned them to preach the Gospel, and one of the signs of true faith would be *casting out demons.*

> *He said to them, "Go into all the world and preach the good news to all creation. Whoever believes and is baptized will be saved, but whoever does not believe will be condemned. And these signs will accompany those who believe: In my name they will drive out demons; they will speak in new tongues;..." Mark 16:14-17*

Another of these signs is *speaking in tongues.* If *speaking in tongues* is a normal expression today, then *casting out demons* is also normal for today. Where these signs fail to appear there must be a faith problem that is usually a result of false teaching on these matters.

---

[3] *Cross Reference: Mark 3:15, 6:13, Matthew 10:8*

Deliverance is an Aspect of Salvation

Deliverance ministry is one aspect of the total salvation that Jesus purchased at His Cross. This salvation includes all God's provision for human need. The Greek word that is translated *saved* is a form of the Greek word *sozo*. This Greek word is also translated in the Gospels in other ways such as *healed, made whole, delivered* or *set free*. When Jesus cast out a demon, he occasionally said. *Your faith has set you free (sozo).* In other words, salvation is more than just being saved from hell. Salvation is healing and deliverance from evil spirits as well.

Deliverance is Salvation from Evil Spirits

Deliverance is God's salvation from evil spirits, and deliverance was purchased by Jesus on the Cross. This is complete and forever finished. Deliverance is received by faith just like salvation from sin, the Baptism in the Holy Spirit or healing. This explains why Christians are sometimes afflicted by demons. Not all believers are automatically experiencing, in all aspects, what Christ did for them on the Cross. Believers fail to appropriate these provisions of salvation out of misdiagnosis of their real need for deliverance, or failure to meet the conditions for receiving. Deliverance or healing is not automatically received when a believer receives Christ. Deliverance is not normally received because of a single one-time prayer either. By persistent and confident warfare prayer, believers apply the defeat of the enemy through faith in the Cross of Christ, and the Holy Spirit will produce a deliverance.

Deliverance for Christians

Deliverance ministry is normally for those who have responded in faith to the gospel of the kingdom and have made Jesus Christ the Lord of their lives. This means that many who need deliverance are not being overwhelmed by demonic power. Their deliverance needs may only exist in one or two areas. Of course, this goes against many people's impressions of deliverance ministry. Hollywood's distorted presentations of deliverance in movies, and some ministries' videotaped public deliverance sessions have given the false impression that anyone with a deliverance need is being overwhelmed by demons. The truth is that while a few people need extensive deliverance, most believers may only need a little.

There are occasions where deliverance is accomplished in the life of someone so seriously afflicted by demons that they are unable to respond to the gospel. However, this is the rare exception rather than the rule. Scripture warns that these spirits will re-enter the *empty house* if it is not filled with Christ. Deliverance belongs to those who in faith are coming to the Lord. Deliverance is the *children's bread*. Believers alone have the right of deliverance from demons. The devil has a legal claim on unbelievers.

Possessed, Oppressed or Obsessed?

Much confusion has arisen in the English speaking Church over the unfortunate use of the English words *possessed*, *obsessed* and *oppressed* to translate the New

Testament Greek verb *diamonizominoi*. [4] The Greek noun *diamon* is normally and properly transliterated *demon* in all modern versions of the Bible. Therefore, the Greek verb above is simply the verb version of the noun *demon*. This Greek verb should be rendered as *demonized* or *to be affected by a demon*. Although translators and interpreters have often used the words *possession, obsession* and *oppression,* these English words are not really supported by this Greek verb. This has caused a great deal of confusion in the Church on this matter. The actual Greek verb does not even imply a certain level of control or reveal whether the demon is inside the person or outside.

Several other phrases are used much less often to describe the condition of a person with a demon. One phrase means *to have an unclean spirit.*[5] Another phrase means to be *with* or *in an unclean spirit.*[6] Sometimes translators have improperly inserted the word *possessed* in these passages as well, even though they do not contain the Greek verb that actually means *demonized.*

It is misleading to say that a Christian can never be *possessed* by evil spirits. Certainly, the Christian is never completely controlled or owned by evil spirits, which is implied by the word *possessed*. God owns the true Christian. However, a demon may affect or *demonize* one or many areas of the life of a Christian. This will result in repeated defeat and failure of the Christian in particular

---

[4]To be *demonized. (diamonizominoi)* Matthew 4:24, 8:16, 8:28, 8:33, 9:32, Mark 5:15, 5:16, 5:18, 9:17, Luke 8:36
[5]To *have an unclean spirit.* Matthew 11:18, Mark 7:25, Luke 8:27
[6]To be *with (*or *in) an unclean spirit.* Mark 1:23, 5:2

areas of behavior, attitudes and possibly sickness. This _demonized_ Christian normally is not fully aware of just what is the real source of his problem. Since God owns the Christian, a demon is _an illegal tenant on God's property._ This _illegal tenant_ is _legally evicted_ by the exercise of authoritative faith of believers in the name of Jesus. This book now turns its attention to the specific incidents of Christ healing through deliverance ministry.

Christ Delivers a Boy from Demonic Seizures

This particular event in the life of Christ and His disciples reveals a great deal concerning supernatural ministry. This is one of the few situations in the New Testament where an apparent failure in ministry occurs. In this case, the failure does not concern Christ but His disciples. However, Christ's explanation of the failure to His disciples is highly instructive to those of us seeking to minister in the supernatural power of God. This passage is found in Chapter 17 of Matthew's Gospel. The Gospel of Mark, Chapter 9, also has the same story.

> _And when they came to the multitude, a man came up to Him, falling on his knees before Him, and saying, "Lord, have mercy on my son, for he is a lunatic, and is very ill; for he often falls into the fire, and often into the water. "And I brought him to Your disciples, and they could not cure him." And Jesus answered and said, "O unbelieving and perverted generation, how long shall I be with you? How long shall I put up with you? Bring him here to Me." And Jesus rebuked him, and the demon came out of him, and the boy was cured at once. Then the_

> *disciples came to Jesus privately and said, "Why could we not cast it out?" And He said to them, "Because of the littleness of your faith; for truly I say to you, if you have faith as a mustard seed, you shall say to this mountain, 'Move from here to there,' and it shall move; and nothing shall be impossible to you. {But this kind does not go out except by prayer and fasting.}" Matthew 17:14-21*

This passage has similarities with another "failure" in ministry that was previously discussed. Later in this chapter, Christ's limitations in His hometown is compared and contrasted with this event. This discussion begins with a description of the situation of the afflicted child.

- *And when they came to the multitude, a man came up to Him, falling on his knees before Him, and saying, "Lord, have mercy on my son, for he is a lunatic, and is very ill; for he often falls into the fire, and often into the water. "*

This father seeks help from Christ for his ill son. The description of the boy is not very clear since there is no longer a medical condition called *lunacy*. However, *lunacy* is a rather indirect translation from the Greek word. The Latin word *luna* means *moon*. (For example, *lunar* means pertaining to the moon.) A literal translation of the Greek into English would be *moon-smitten*. In other words, this child is described as being affected negatively by the moon. However, the real problem is that this child has a demon that causes him to have seizures in dangerous places where he could be serious harmed or killed. This has been often thought of as the condition of epilepsy, but actually could have been something else.

- *And I brought him to Your disciples, and they could not cure him." And Jesus answered and said, "O unbelieving and perverted generation, how long shall I be with you? How long shall I put up with you?*

The father explained to Christ that His disciples could not deal with his son's dangerous seizures. Christ strong reaction to this failure on the part of His disciples is revealing. Christ says that they are *unbelieving and perverted*. The implication is that if they were not *unbelieving and perverted* they could have dealt with the boy's illness.

The Greek word for *unbelieving* is a form of the word for *faith* simply in a negative form. The Greek word translated *perverted* means literally *twisted* or *distorted*. Christ says, in effect, that they cannot deal with this situation because they lack *faith* and have character and attitudes that seriously vary from God's norm for humanity. In other words, the disciples should have been able to deal with this situation if their faith and character had been what the Father desires for humanity.

This passage reveals that the will of the Father is not the obstacle affecting this child's healing. The obstacle to the healing that is revealed here is a human deficiency of faith and character. (Thank God that He is willing to help us correct these limiting conditions.) Christ, however, had no problem dealing with this boy's illness.

- *Bring him here to Me." And Jesus rebuked him, and the demon came out of him, and the boy was cured at once.*

    Jesus cast out the demon that was causing this boy's illness and injuries. This malevolent being, a demon, was obviously trying to harm or kill the boy by causing him to fall into water to drown him or into fires to burn him. Christ, without any hesitation about the will of the Father, dealt with the demon and the boy's illness was *cured.*

- *Then the disciples came to Jesus privately and said, "Why could we not cast it out?"*

    This is an appropriate question from the disciples of Christ. They had already experienced some ministry on occasions that *duplicated* Christ's ministry. They had been commissioned by Christ to heal the sick and cast out demons as they preached the gospel of the Kingdom of God. (This is recorded in Matthew, Chapter 10.) *So, why had they failed in this situation?* Christ answers their question very directly.

- *And He said to them, "Because of the littleness of your faith; for truly I say to you, if you have faith as a mustard seed, you shall say to this mountain, 'Move from here to there,' and it shall move; and nothing shall be impossible to you.*

    The disciples had failed to deal with the boy's need because of the *littleness of their faith.* Christ elaborates on the need for faith in these matters by telling them (and us)

170

that only a small amount of faith is necessary to accomplish great things. The mustard seed is practically microscopic. Christ could not have used a smaller object known to His hearers to illustrate the small amount of faith necessary to accomplish the boy's deliverance. However, Christ's point here is that the disciples did not even have even that much faith in God, and that is why they had failed. This is the second time in this situation that Christ has mentioned _unbelief_ or _a lack of faith_.

Christ tells them that a microscopically small amount of faith will cause _nothing to be impossible_ to them. In this context, the humanly impossible things that would become possible would be the healing and deliverance of people with mental conditions, injuries and sicknesses.

The theological idea that the Father's will is a problem in healing is not present in this account. There is no problem with the Father being willing to deliver this boy. The real problem is on the human side of the equation. Faith is again the issue. Christ says even the impossible will be possible to those who believe.

This situation is remarkably similar to one of the general description that was studied in the early chapters of this book. That particular situation was Christ ministering in His own hometown, where He was unable to minister at the same level of the supernatural as in other places. In that situation, the text tells us that the reason for Christ's partial "failure" was the _unbelief_ of the people in His hometown. In this passage, the failure of the disciples of Jesus is attributed to _unbelief_ as well. Christ reveals that the solution is faith.

- _{"But this kind does not go out except by prayer and fasting.}_

The reason for this verse being in parenthesis is that it is a textual variant. A textual variant is a word, phrase or text that _varies_ in the existing ancient copies of the books of the New Testament. In other words, some of the existing ancient manuscripts have this verse and some do not. However, this verse does not change anything substantially, except to say to us that some demons may be strong enough to resist ordinary faith in Christ. However, no one should ever despair that their situation requires more faith than they presently have. Greater faith in Christ is easily obtainable. What is needed in an unusually difficult kind of situation is faith in Christ made strong by prayer and fasting.

The Gerasene Demoniac

Sometimes this man has been called the Gaderene Demoniac. This story is found in all three Synoptic Gospels. It is included in this book because it concerns a condition of insanity. The man in this story was insane because he had so many demons. Here is the story from the Gospel of Luke:

> _...And when He had come out onto the land (the Geresenes), He was met by a certain man from the city who was possessed with demons; and who had not put on any clothing for a long time, and was not_

living in a house, but in the tombs. And seeing Jesus, he cried out and fell before Him, and said in a loud voice, "What do I have to do with You, Jesus, Son of the Most High God? I beg You, do not torment me." For He had been commanding the unclean spirit to come out of the man. For it had seized him many times; and he was bound with chains and shackles and kept under guard; and yet he would burst his fetters and be driven by the demon into the desert. And Jesus asked him, "What is your name?" And he said, "Legion"; for many demons had entered him. And they were entreating Him not to command them to depart into the abyss. Now there was a herd of many swine feeding there on the mountain; and the demons entreated Him to permit them to enter the swine. And He gave them permission. And the demons came out from the man and entered the swine; and the herd rushed down the steep bank into the lake, and were drowned... and they (the observers) came to Jesus, and found the man from whom the demons had gone out, sitting down at the feet of Jesus, clothed and in his right mind... And those who had seen it reported to them how the man who was demon-possessed had been made well. Luke 8:27-36 (edited for purposes of brevity)

This long passage gives us a number of matters to consider.

- *...And when He had come out onto the land (the Geresenes), He was met by a certain man from the city* *who was possessed with demons; and who had not put on any clothing for a long time, and was not living in a house, but in the tombs.*

Christ met a man that was quite insane. The insanity in this case was being produced by demons. The account gives us some specific details about this man and his behavior. For instance, the account tells us that he was from the city. The account tells us that he was naked and he had been that way for a long period as a result of his own bizarre behavior rather than poverty or some other reason. He also apparently could have lived in a house but was living among the dead in the tombs, probably caves in the region. Things were about to change now that this insane man encountered Christ.

- *And seeing Jesus, he cried out and fell before Him, and said in a loud voice...*

This demonized man has a strong reaction to Christ's presence. He cries out, falls down before Christ and then begins to speak to Christ with a loud voice. In the beginning of this story, it seems that Christ is dealing with one demon. However as the story unfolds, the reader learns that there are many demons. After the complete context of this conversation is considered, there is no doubt that the man is not speaking. Instead, the demons in him are speaking through him to Christ.

- *What do I have to do with You, Jesus, Son of the Most High God?*

The demons recognize *exactly* with whom they are dealing. They know Christ's name. They know that Jesus is the incarnate Son of God. They know that they have no legitimate relationship with Christ. The question that the demons ask reveals their desire to know what Christ wants from them. The next two phrases put this question into a clearer context.

- *...I beg You, do not torment me.*

The demons ask Christ not to torment them. How was Christ tormenting them? Christ was commanding the spirit to leave the man.

- *For He had been commanding the unclean spirit to come out of the man.*

This phrase reveals that the man's reaction in the beginning was a result of Christ commanding the unclean spirit to come out. This action of Christ was *tormenting* the spirits in this man. For those who think that Christ always accomplished everything He wanted at once, this passage is a contradiction. This passage reveals that Christ had commanded the spirits to come out of this man *without initial success.* The unclean spirits remained in this man *after* Christ had commanded them to come out. This is another place where Christ worked with someone through a spiritual need until they were healed or delivered. If one wishes a Christ-like ministry, willingness to work through a need until the Father's answer in Christ is revealed is essential. This particular man's condition would have been very difficult for anyone to say that it was doing him some mysterious good.

- *For it (the demon) had seized him many times; and he was bound with chains and shackles and kept under guard; and yet he would burst his fetters and be driven by the demon into the desert.*

The way that this portion of the text reads indicates that there were moments of sanity for this man when demonic influence was not entirely obvious. However, the demons *seized* the man *many times*. The description of the attempt to restrain this man reveals that there was concern either for the safety of the man or for others. The fact that the demons would drive him into the desert meant that his own life was in danger. Mark's version of this story adds an additional detail that says that the man was *gashing himself with stones*[7]. Whether this was suicidal behavior or just self-abuse is not clear. Nevertheless, eventually this kind of behavior would have shortened or ended this man's life.

The man's ability to break free from *chains*, *shackles* and guards reveals demonically inspired supernatural strength. This is common in persons with many demons. This incredible strength and his unpredictable behavior would have made him a danger to those around him.

---

[7] Mark 5:5

- *And Jesus asked him, "What is your name?" And he said, "Legion"; for many demons had entered him.*

This book is not attempting to teach on demons and deliverance except where the passages apply to the healing of various conditions. However, this passage does give important information about demons and their nature that should not be ignored. For instance, Christ *assumed* that the demon that he was dealing with would have a name. Additionally, the passage reveals that the demons have knowledge of Christ's authority over them.

- *And they were entreating Him not to command them to depart into the abyss.*

The demons knew that Christ could command them to leave the man. They had previously resisted coming out and were apparently trying to bargain with Christ before coming out. An attempt at bargaining is common in deliverance ministry as well. These demons were particularly distressed at the thought that Christ might send them to the *abyss*[8]. The abyss is the place of imprisonment of the devil for a thousand years according to the Revelation. The demons' knowledge of this place and Christ's potential to send them there is interesting, but has little to do with healing. So this matter will not be pursued any further. Christ does not comment on the matter of the

---

[8] Sometimes translated as "the bottomless pit" found in Luke 8:31, Romans 10:7, Revelation 9:1-2, 11, 11:7, 17:8, 20:1, 3

abyss but casts out the demons and actually fulfills their request to enter a herd of swine.

- *Now there was a herd of many swine feeding there on the mountain; and the demons entreated Him to permit them to enter the swine. And He gave them permission. And the demons came out from the man and entered the swine; and the herd rushed down the steep bank into the lake, and were drowned...*

Knowing that Christ had authority to cast them out, it appears that the demons reluctantly but *voluntarily* left the man and entered the swine. Perhaps Christ allowed this to occur because it was better for the man than if the demons had continued to resist. In any case, the demons left the insane man and entered the swine. The passage reveals that the swine drowned in the lake after the demons entered them. The focus, however, is not upon the demons or the swine but upon the previously demonized man.

- *and they (the observers) came to Jesus, and found the man from whom the demons had gone out, sitting down at the feet of Jesus, clothed and in his right mind...*

The man was in his *right mind* as a result of the demons leaving him. The man was clothed and appropriately was sitting at the feet of his Deliverer. This passage indicates that this man's bizarre behavior, his great strength and violence, his self-mutilation, his suicidal gestures, and his public nudity were entirely caused by demonic activity.

- *And those who had seen it reported to them how the man who was demon-possessed had been made well.*

This man had been *made well.* The phrase *made well* is a form of the Greek word *sozo* in the Greek manuscripts. This is the word that is alternatively translated as *saved, healed, delivered, made well, made whole, set free* and a variety of other ways. The noun form of this word is normally translated as *salvation.* In other words, this demonized and insane man experienced *salvation* in the form of deliverance from evil spirits.

The Blind and Mute Man

There are a number of accounts of Christ healing the blind. Several of them indicate that demons were the reason for the blindness of the person that He healed. In this particular case, the demonic activity in this man's life was causing both blindness and an inability to speak.

> *Then there was brought to Him a demon-possessed man who was blind and dumb, and He healed him, so that the dumb man spoke and saw. And all the multitudes were amazed, and began to say, "This man cannot be the Son of David, can he?" But when the Pharisees heard it, they said, "This man casts out demons only by Beelzebul the ruler of the demons." Matthew 12:22-24*

This passage has a few new thoughts to consider:

- *Then there was brought to Him a demon-possessed man who was blind and dumb...*

179

Performing Miracles and Healing

The man was blind and dumb because of demonic activity. Demonic activity apparently can cause a variety of serious disabilities, sicknesses and afflictions. It is unlikely however, that anyone knew that demons were the source of this man's disabilities. They probably came to know the true source of this man's problems after Christ ministered to him. Of course, no one would suggest now that somehow these demons were producing a mysterious good from God in these disabilities in this man's life. However, it would be possible today for someone to suggest it if they were ignorant that the actual cause of a blind or mute person's condition was demonic activity. In other words, today much displacement of responsibility for illness occurs. God is sometimes given credit for doing a mysterious work for good in a person's disabilities when actually a hidden destructive work of demons is taking place.

The record that this man was *brought to Him* is consistent with the blindness of the man. This does not reveal anything specifically concerning *who believed* that Christ could help. The afflicted man might have heard of Christ and somehow communicated that he wanted to be taken to Christ. However, it is much more likely that a caring friend or relative *believed* that Christ could help him and brought him to Christ. In any case, the action reveals that someone *believed* that Christ could help him.

- *... and He healed him...*

The blind and mute man was *healed*. Often the words for healing are applied in the New Testament when deliverance occurs from evil spirits causing a condition or sickness. Therefore, any teaching on healing is incomplete if that teaching fails to deal with demonic activity producing sickness and disability.

- *...so that the dumb man spoke and saw.*

The demonized man's healing was complete. He was able to speak and see immediately after Christ dealt with the demons.

- *And all the multitudes were amazed, and began to say, "This man cannot be the Son of David, can he?"*

The effects of this healing deliverance were apparent. The masses were *amazed*. The masses began to question if Jesus might not be the predicted Messiah, who would be a descendent of King David. In other words, faith in Christ began to be inspired in those who were aware of this man's healing deliverance.

Evangelism is accelerated because miracles inspire faith in Christ. As the Church approaches the end of the age and the final harvest of souls, evangelism will need healings and deliverance such as this one. However, not everyone will believe at the end of the age even if they see the miracles. In fact, some powerless religious leaders will become accusers and attribute the works of Christ to the devil. If Christ could not avoid accusation, neither will His Church. The spirit of the Pharisee was found then and is present now and will be present in the future.

- *But when the Pharisees heard it, they said, "This man casts out demons only by Beelzebul the ruler of the demons."*

Earlier in this passage, the demonized man was described as being *healed*. The words of the Pharisees reveal that Christ must have *cast out* the demons causing this man's condition since that kind of ministry was what they were specifically criticizing. In other words, sometimes in those cases where demons are causing a sickness, condition or disability, the New Testament may describe deliverance from the demons as a *healing* or as *casting out demons*.

The Syro-Phoenician Woman's Daughter

This story, found in Matthew's Gospel, reveals a situation that involves some unique elements that are of great interest to anyone seeking to consistently perform healing and miracles. It is included because at the end of the story, Matthew describes this deliverance from evil spirits as a *healing*.

The situation involves a child who has specific needs for deliverance from evil spirits. Of additional interest is the fact that this case involves the faith of someone else for the demonized child.

And Jesus...withdrew into district of Tyre and Sidon. And behold, a Canaanite woman came out from that region, and began to cry out, saying, "Have mercy on me, O Lord, Son of David; my daughter is cruelly demon-possessed." But He did _not answer her a word. And His disciples came to Him and kept asking Him, saying, "Send her away, for she is shouting out after us." But He answered and said, "I was sent only to the lost sheep of the house of Israel." But she came and began to bow down before Him, saying, "Lord, help me!" And He answered and said, "It is not good to take the children's bread and throw it to the dogs." But she said, "Yes, Lord; but even the dogs feed on the crumbs which fall from their masters' table." Then Jesus answered and said to her, "O woman, your faith is great; be it done for you as you wish." And her daughter was healed at once. Matthew 15:21-28_

The story takes place just after a conflict with the Pharisees and Scribes. This may explain why the passage says that Christ _withdrew_ into the district of Tyre and Sidon. This region is outside of the normal borders of Israel. Perhaps, Christ was there to have a time of rest for Himself and His disciples.

- _And Jesus...withdrew into the district of Tyre and Sidon. And behold, a Canaanite woman came out from that region, and began to cry out, saying, "Have mercy on me, O Lord, Son of David; my daughter is cruelly demon-possessed."_

The Canaanite woman in this story is described as being very vocal about her daughter's need. She certainly believed that Christ could help her daughter. This is revealed in her behavior. She also addressed Christ with a messianic title that was seen earlier in this chapter. She called Christ the *Son of David*. She also asked for *mercy,* which is repeatedly heard from those who receive healing from Christ. Christ's reaction to her is somewhat different than some of the other descriptions of His healing ministry.

- *But He did not answer her a word. And His disciples came to Him and kept asking Him, saying, "Send her away, for she is shouting out after us." But He answered and said, "I was sent only to the lost sheep of the house of Israel."*

The disciples ask Christ to do something about this gentile woman. Apparently, her persistence, revealed in her shouting at Christ and His disciples, began to bother them. However, Christ reveals that the reason He has not helped this woman is due to the limitations of His *call*. His *call* was to the people of Israel and she was not Jewish. In other words, Christ understood that it was possible for Him to unwisely spend His time and effort outside of His basic call to the Nation of Israel. Christ was presently in a region that was outside His call and inhabited primarily by gentile people.

- *But she came and began to bow down before Him, saying, "Lord, help me!" And He answered and said, "It is not good to take the children's bread and throw it to the dogs."*

More than anything else, this passage reveals a continuing persistence on the part of this woman. She would not be denied. However, Christ again revealed that His ministry to Israel was His primary concern. Christ described His ministry as *the children's bread*. God had prepared the *children* of Israel to receive the early ministry of Messiah. On the other hand, the gentile nations had not received the same sort of preparation. Christ was saying that if He were to focus His ministry on the gentile nations, it would be like taking food prepared for the *children* of a family and giving it to the *dogs* instead. Christ explained that responding to this woman would be a potential misuse of the spiritual resources that God had given to Him.

- *But she said, "Yes, Lord; but even the dogs feed on the crumbs which fall from their masters' table."*

The woman, however, is not deterred by Christ's explanation of why He will not help her. Instead, she uses Christ's own logic and illustration to say that, even if there are limitations to Christ's ministry, there is such an abundance of *bread* that some is likely to end up as *crumbs* that will feed the dogs. In other words, this woman has argued that all that Christ must provide for her is a *crumb;* and consequently, there will be no loss of His focus on the children of Israel. The children will be fed anyway, even if a few crumbs end up with the dogs. Christ has an obvious change of heart due to this woman's persistence.

- *Then Jesus answered and said to her, "O woman, your faith is great; be it done for you as you wish." And her daughter was healed at once.*

Christ sees this woman's persistence as *great faith*. She was not willing to receive these negative answers from Christ. In fact, despite Christ's early disregard for her cries,

Christ. In fact, despite Christ's early disregard for her cries, and His twice explaining to her why He would not help her, she persisted and received what she wished from the Father. Her daughter was healed.

This story has strong implications to consider on the matter of the will of the Father. This story shows a possible limitation of the will of God in a matter of healing or deliverance. However, the limitation is specifically revealed as pertaining to the call of Christ to Israel and not any other reason. In other words, the child in this story was not suffering from demonic power because some mysterious good was happening, but simply because Christ was not called to her people and region. However, persistent faith overcame even those limitations.

Great faith allowed this woman to receive something from which she would have normally been excluded. Her timing was simply wrong. Christ's ministry had not yet been released in and through His Church. It was then limited to His person and the small band of His disciples. However, all these limitations were overcome by overcoming faith. Thankfully, the day has come where Christ's ministry to this region and this race has come through His Church.

The Mute Demoniac

This is the second story of someone being mute caused by demonic activity. In the earlier account in this chapter, the man was also blind. Here is the story:

> *And as they were going out, behold, a dumb man, demon-possessed, was brought to Him. And after*

186

the demon was cast out, the dumb man spoke; and the multitudes marveled, saying, "Nothing like this was ever seen in Israel." But the Pharisees were saying, "He casts out the demons by the ruler of the demons." Matthew 9:32-34

This story occurs in a chapter full of healing, deliverance and even a resurrection. It occurs as Christ and His disciples leave a house where the two blind men were healed.

- *And as they were going out, behold, a dumb man, demon-possessed, was brought to Him.*

The man's condition of being mute was being caused by demons. Someone brought this man to Christ to help him. Obviously, whoever brought him must have believed that Christ could help him.

- *And after the demon was cast out, the dumb man spoke...*

Immediately the man's condition was cured after the demon was cast out. The man could speak. This caused quite a reaction in those that observed this deliverance.

- *...and the multitudes marveled, saying, "Nothing like this was ever seen in Israel." But the Pharisees were saying, "He casts out the demons by the ruler of the demons."*

There were two opposing reactions to the help that this man got. The first was that the common people *marveled* and were obviously positively affected. The second was that the religious leaders began to criticize and attributed the healing to the devil. These are the typical reactions today. Either people will be encouraged and positively respond to the grace of God being demonstrated, or they will become critical and somehow devalue the healing or the person who is doing healing ministry.

Woman Bound for Eighteen Years

Christ encountered a woman in a synagogue who had an affliction caused by a demon. Here is the first half of this story:

> *And He was teaching in one of the synagogues on the Sabbath. And behold, there was a woman who for eighteen years had had a sickness caused by a spirit; and she was bent double, and could not straighten up at all. And when Jesus saw her, He called her over and said to her, "Woman, you are freed from your sickness." And He laid His hands upon her; and immediately she was made erect again, and began glorifying God. Luke 13:10-13*

Christ's ministry carried Him into a synagogue where he encountered a woman who had been sick for eighteen years as a result of the work of a demon.

- *And He was teaching in one of the synagogues on the Sabbath. And behold, there was a woman who for eighteen years had had a sickness caused by a spirit;*

and she was bent double, and could not straighten up at all.

The passage does not say what the sickness was, but it caused a specific symptom of her being bent double with an inability to stand straight up. Perhaps she had severe arthritis or some other similar condition. It is likely that neither she nor anyone else understood that a spirit was causing her physical problem. In fact, she was probably going about her normal Sabbath activities when Christ called her over.

Deliverance needs may be disguised behind normal symptoms of disease or conditions. They remain disguised partly because of the confusion caused by the use of the word *possessed* in the English versions of the New Testament. Many people fail to recognize deliverance needs because they think that the person must be fully controlled by demons in order to need deliverance. This is not the case. Sometimes people need deliverance from a few spirits that are afflicting them in a particular area. (For those who need additional information on deliverance ministry, there are excellent resources available in most Christian bookstores for learning about this kind of ministry.)

- *And when Jesus saw her, He called her over and said to her, "Woman, you are freed from your sickness." And He laid His hands upon her; and immediately she was made erect again, and began glorifying God.*

Performing Miracles and Healing

Christ boldly healed this woman by laying His hands on her. Despite the fact that her sickness was being caused by a spirit, Christ healed her in much the same way that he healed in situations where a demon is not revealed. In other words, many times the laying hands on a person in faith may produce deliverance from evil spirits without a protracted battle. However, occasionally a protracted ministry is necessary to accomplish deliverance and healing. In this case, however, Christ accomplished deliverance easily much like He healed the sick. However, Christ used language that indicated that deliverance had occurred. Christ said to her that *Woman, you are freed from your sickness.* The fact that Christ said she was *freed* rather than *healed* indicated that a deliverance rather than healing was taking place. The fact that the woman was *immediately* able to stand upright also reveals that the spirit causing the sickness was then gone. The reaction of the leader of the Synagogue to this deliverance is interesting:

> *And the synagogue official, indignant because Jesus had healed on the Sabbath, began saying to the multitude in response, "There are six days in which work should be done; therefore come during them and get healed, and not on the Sabbath day." But the Lord answered him and said, "You hypocrites, does not each of you on the Sabbath untie his ox or his donkey from the stall, and lead him away to water him? And this woman, a daughter of Abraham as she is, whom Satan has bound for eighteen long years, should she not have been released from this bond on the Sabbath day?" And as He said this, all His opponents were being humiliated; and the entire multitude was rejoicing*

190

over all the glorious things being done by Him. Luke 13:14-17

The second part of this story reveals that the Synagogue official was critical of Christ healing this woman on the Sabbath. The official acted as if healing were a violation of religious law and therefore of the will of God.

- *And the synagogue official, indignant because Jesus had healed on the Sabbath, began saying to the multitude in response, "There are six days in which work should be done; therefore come during them and get healed, and not on the Sabbath day."*

Similar public and private reactions are found to healing today. Some misguided religious leaders treat those who heal the sick as if they were doing something wrong. This synagogue official reacted as if God was not involved in healing this woman. He reacted as if the healing could wait for another day. He was accusing Christ of violating the Sabbath prohibitions and therefore of wrongdoing.

The synagogue official said *get healed.* This indicates that from the perspective of the onlookers, Christ had simply laid His hands on the woman and then she was able to stand upright. In other words, the demon probably was not evident to the onlookers. They simply saw a healing. Christ on the other hand knew that there was a evil spirit involved.

Christ answered the accusation of the synagogue official that He had done something wrong by using a simple comparison.

- *But the Lord answered him and said, "You hypocrites, does not each of you on the Sabbath untie his ox or his donkey from the stall, and lead him away to water him?*

Christ drew a comparison from the normal care of domestic animals. Christ argues that the normal care of domestic animals on the Sabbath obviously does not violate the Sabbath. If this is true, the supernatural care of this woman demonstrated by her healing and deliverance cannot violate the Sabbath. A powerful truth emerges from Christ's comparison. *Healing and deliverance is normal care for a believer in the same way that watering is for farm animals.* If watering is a necessary action and compassionate response to a farm animal, then healing and deliverance are necessary actions and compassionate responses to people. Christ then says:

- *"And this woman, a daughter of Abraham as she is, whom Satan has bound for eighteen long years, should she not have been released from this bond on the Sabbath day?"*

Christ could have avoided criticism by waiting another day to minister to this woman. However, the Lord was unwilling to have this woman suffer any longer despite what His critics might think about Him healing on the Sabbath.

Healing and Demonic Activity

Christ said that _Satan has bound_ this woman. Earlier in the account, the passage revealed that a _spirit_ was causing her sickness. Christ was not dealing with Satan himself. He was dealing with one of Satan's low-level, subordinate spirits. The fact that Christ said _Satan has bound_ this woman reveals that Satan's kingdom is organized and is causing sickness and other problems in humanity through evil spirits. In other words, Christ credited Satan with this woman's sickness because, ultimately, Satan had commanded his subordinate spirits to do this kind of harm to humanity.

If sickness was doing this woman some mysterious good during the time that she suffered, it is hard to see in this account. In fact, Christ said that the eighteen years were eighteen _long_ years. Christ described what she experienced as being _released from this bond._ Christ released her from the torture of _bondage_ and captivity to an evil spirit.

Today because of extreme popular teaching about the value of suffering by sickness, a person afflicted by the power of an evil spirit might be taught that their suffering is actually God doing a mysterious work within their lives. Misdiagnosis of the actual cause of conditions creates confusion and doubt. This kind of misdiagnosis of the source of the suffering of people is common today. However, when the ministry of Christ is examined fully, and the will of the Father is seen clearly in that examination, healing and deliverance begin to displace the false religious teaching. The mental strongholds that oppose Christ-like healing and deliverance begin to crumble, as Christ becomes the foundation of Christian teaching and ministry.

- *And as He said this, all His opponents were being humiliated; and the entire multitude was rejoicing over all the glorious things being done by Him.*

The common people saw Christ's ministry as full of glorious things. On the other hand, the religious leaders who opposed Him failed to see this and were being humiliated. When Christ-like healing and miracle ministry is resisted the inevitable result is humiliation for those who are resisting. Unfortunately, when leaders fail to humbly equip themselves in the supernatural arena, they may ultimately resist out of insecurity and misunderstanding of those who are equipped. This is to the detriment of the Kingdom of God, the people of God and themselves. Humiliation will be the result of resisting the supernatural equipping of the saints for the final harvest at the end of the age. Thankfully, the majority of leaders will sense the shortness of the time and humbly allow themselves to be equipped to demonstrate Christ-like ministry in the earth.

The Healing of Various Women

In Luke Chapter 8, a passage exists that seems to be partly general and partly specific. It addresses an unnamed *many others* in a general way and specifically names three of the women who were healed by Christ. It is included with the specific accounts because it does address some women by name. It also has some things to say about demonic activity and sickness.

Healing and Demonic Activity

> *...and also some women who had been healed of evil spirits and sicknesses: Mary who was called Magdalene, from whom seven demons had gone out, and Joanna the wife of Chuza, Herod's steward, and Susanna, and many others who were contributing to their support out of their private means. Luke 8:2-3*

From this short passage, several things are noteworthy:

* *...and also some women who had been healed of evil spirits and sicknesses...*

Luke uses the general term *healed* to describe deliverance from *evil spirits* and healing of *sicknesses.* Luke's usage of *healed of evil spirits* may indicate that these evil spirits were causing sickness in these women. However, since Luke has separated *evil spirits* and *sicknesses,* this substantiates the fact that *all* sickness is *not directly caused* by evil spirits. In fact, as this book has attempted to analyze the various passages concerning healing, it is evident that about one-quarter of the recorded specific healing events in Christ's ministry openly reveal the work of demons causing sickness or a disabling condition. In other words, any ministry wishing to function as Christ did in bringing healing ministry to people must be willing and able to deal with demonic activity when it is discovered.

~9~

Christ Heals Disability & Injury

The Deaf and Mute Man in Decapolis

While some deafness is the result of demonic activity, the Gospels also reveal this healing of deafness that does not mention demonic activity. Here is the story that is found only in the Gospel of Mark:

And they brought to Him one who was deaf and spoke with difficulty, and they entreated Him to lay His hand upon him. And He took him aside from the multitude by himself, and put His fingers into his ears, and after spitting, He touched his tongue with the saliva; and looking up to heaven with a deep sigh, He said to him, "Ephphatha!" that is, "Be opened!" And his ears were opened, and the impediment of his tongue was removed, and he began speaking plainly. And He gave them orders not to tell anyone; but the more He ordered them, the more widely they continued to proclaim it. And they were utterly astonished, saying, "He has done all things well; He makes even the deaf to hear, and the dumb to speak." Mark 7:32-37

Christ's healing of this deaf and partially mute man has a number of points to teach concerning healing:

- *And they brought to Him one who was deaf and spoke with difficulty, and they entreated Him to lay His hand upon him.*

Christ's reputation as a healer must have reached the family and friends of this blind and partially mute man. They brought him to Christ and wanted Christ to *lay His hands upon him*. This shows again that Christ's most often used method of healing was the *laying on of hands*. Christ must have used it so often that everyone expected this man to be healed when Christ used this method.

- *And He took him aside from the multitude by himself...*

Christ had on several occasions changed the location of someone before healing them. This time, Christ took the man aside from the multitude before healing him. This could mean that Christ and the man were alone. It could mean that Christ's disciples were also present. There are some indicators later in this passage that strongly suggest the disciples were present. The reasons for removing the man from the multitude are not entirely obvious. Changing the circumstance before healing someone is common in Christ's ministry. Since the healing of hearing was involved, perhaps Christ needed a quiet place, a controlled environment, to minister so He could determine more precisely what was happening with the man. Perhaps, Christ needed to be able to hear the man speak and to determine how well the man was hearing. The noise of a multitude would interfere with that.

- _and put His fingers into his ears, and after spitting, He touched his tongue with the saliva; and looking up to heaven with a deep sigh, He said to him, "Ephphatha!" that is, "Be opened!"_

Putting fingers into a deaf person's ears is a form of the _laying on of hands_. Christ's command for the ears to _open_ is not unusual either. Christ uses commands in several healings, particularly when a demon is involved. In this case, the phrase, _looking up to heaven with a deep sigh_, reveals that Christ was in silent communion with the Father. Perhaps the unusual methodology of touching the man's tongue with His saliva came as Divine guidance.

- _And his ears were opened, and the impediment of his tongue was removed, and he began speaking plainly._

Christ restored the man's hearing. In the language of the New Testament, _his ears were opened_. This implies that his ears were _closed_ before meeting Christ. This fits with Christ's command to the ears to _open_. The rest of the statement indicates that something, an _impediment_, was preventing the man from speaking clearly. The Greek word that is translated _impediment_ is _mogilatos_. This word is a combination of _mogis_ and _laleo_. These words mean respectively _difficulty_ and _speaking_. So all the passage really says is that the *speaking difficulty* was removed. Possibly the man stammered or simply spoke unclearly simply because he could not hear before Christ healed him. In any case, the problem was removed.

- *And He gave them orders not to tell anyone; but the more He ordered them, the more widely they continued to proclaim it.*

The fact that Christ told *them* not to tell anyone probably indicates that the disciples were present. The statement, *but the more He ordered them*, strongly suggests that the disciples were present. Christ not wanting them to tell anyone could also be a reason for removing this man from the multitude. Christ was already dealing with a multitude, He did not want additional publicity. However, Christ was unsuccessful in preventing the publication of this miracle.

- *And they were utterly astonished, saying, "He has done all things well; He makes even the deaf to hear, and the dumb to speak."*

It makes sense that the *they* referred to here is the disciples. The disciples had observed Christ's ministry to all kinds of people with all kinds of problems. Their testimony, *"He has done all things well..."*, indicates that they had been witnesses to Christ's ministry throughout.

This miracle is the tenth of fourteen specific miracles and healings that occur in Mark's Gospel. The last three chapters contain information about the last week of

Christ's life without mentioning a healing.[1] The chapters preceding the last three chapters contain Christ's teaching and a few healings and miracles. In other words, the disciples had already witnessed many miracles and healings. Their testimony was, _"He has done all things well; He makes even the deaf to hear, and the dumb to speak."_

The fact that the disciples knew that Christ had _done all things well_ in the arena of healing suggests they were unaware of Christ failing to get people healed. Opponents of modern healing ministry and those still affected by the teaching of opponents to healing ministry often argue that Christ did not heal everyone who came to Him in faith. They argue this point from a few general passages where Christ is dealing with a multitude. Some of these passages do not say that _all were healed_. Some give no indication about numbers at all. Some passages may say _many_ were healed. This focus on _many_, badly interpreted to mean that some were not healed, is a way of looking for a _theological loophole_.

If it can be established that Christ did not heal everyone who came to Him in faith then a _theological loophole_ is established. This loophole would mean that no one could be sure that Christ would heal even if the needy person has genuine faith. Of course, this approach will undermine faith. In fact, if believers cannot be completely certain of the reliability, the faithfulness of Christ in healing, how can they really _believe_ in Christ as Healer? A

---

[1] Except for Malchus' ear. However, Mark's Gospel does not say that he was healed. Only Luke reveals that Christ healed Malchus.

religious explanation that God is good but will not always heal is not enough. It is *impossible* to put faith in that which is perceived as unpredictable and unreliable. Christians may desperately pray and hope for healing from an unpredictable God. However, believers can only have faith in that which is believed to be always faithful. Thankfully, the disciples reveal to believers today that Christ *did all things well* in matters of healing and miracles. The disciples had seen Christ minister to multitudes, and they were not aware of any failures on His part. When confronted with the multitudes, Christ *did all things well*. Christ faithfully healed all those who came to Him in faith.

The Man at the Sheep Gate Pool

Early in the Gospel of John, Christ ministered healing to a man at a pool of water near the Sheep gate in Jerusalem. The apostle John is the only Gospel writer that records this healing. Here is the first half of the story of this man's healing:

> *Now there is in Jerusalem by the sheep gate a pool, which is called in Hebrew Bethesda, having five porticoes. In these lay a multitude of those who were sick, blind, lame, and withered, {waiting for the moving of the waters; for an angel of the Lord went down at certain seasons into the pool, and stirred up the water; whoever then first, after the stirring up of the water, stepped in was made well from whatever disease with which he was afflicted.}*
> *John 5:2-4*

Christ Heals Disability and Injury

The first half of the story sets the stage for this man's healing. Because John was an eyewitness to this healing, he is able to describe in great detail the location where it occurred. These details are obviously an important part in understanding what happened in this story. The area where the healing happened is called *Bethesda*, which means in Hebrew, *House of Mercy*. Here is John's description of the location of this healing:

- *Now there is in Jerusalem by the sheep gate a pool, which is called in Hebrew Bethesda, having five porticoes. In these lay a multitude of those who were sick, blind, lame, and withered...*

A great number of people needing the mercy of God in healing were waiting near this pool because it had a reputation for occasionally producing a supernatural healing. There were five porticoes or covered porches where these unfortunate people were waiting for healing.

- *{waiting for the moving of the waters; for an angel of the Lord went down at certain seasons into the pool, and stirred up the water; whoever then first, after the stirring up of the water, stepped in was made well from whatever disease with which he was afflicted.}*

The New American Standard has this verse in parenthesis because many of the existing ancient manuscripts of the Gospel of John do not contain this verse. Some have discounted this verse as being valid on that basis or because the verse is unusual and very supernatural. However, since supernatural healing is found throughout the Old Testament, there seems no real reason to doubt that this angelic phenomenon was actually happening. Logic indicates that something must have been happening. There must have been a strong motivation for all these unfortunate and suffering people to gather there. Also the sick man's own words a few verses later confirm that he was waiting for the water to be stirred. That part of the story is found in all manuscripts. Here is the second part of this story:

> *And a certain man was there, who had been thirty-eight years in his sickness. When Jesus saw him lying there, and knew that he had already been a long time in that condition, He said to him, "Do you wish to get well?" The sick man answered Him, "Sir, I have no man to put me into the pool when the water is stirred up, but while I am coming, another steps down before me." Jesus said to him, "Arise, take up your pallet, and walk." And immediately the man became well, and took up his pallet and began to walk. Now it was the Sabbath on that day... Afterward Jesus found him in the temple, and said to him, "Behold, you have become well; do not sin anymore, so that nothing worse may befall you." John 5:5-9, 14*

The account of this healing reveals some important and encouraging points in relationship with the Father's willingness to heal.

● *And a certain man was there, who had been thirty-eight years in his sickness. When Jesus saw him lying there,* _and knew that he had already been a long time in that condition, He said to him, "Do you wish to get well?"_

This man had been sick for thirty-eight years. While the passage does not indicate what was wrong with him, it does reveal that he could not walk. Christ asks the man if he wished to get well. This strongly suggests that the man had adjusted emotionally to his condition. The fact he had been sick for thirty-eight years, however, was not evidence that the Father wanted him sick for some mysterious reason.

- _The sick man answered Him, "Sir, I have no man to put me into the pool when the water is stirred up, but while I am coming, another steps down before me."_

Perhaps the man is explaining his situation, or perhaps he feels sorry for himself. Maybe he had believed, for many years without success, that he would be healed. He complained that he had no one to help him get in the pool. Since only one person at a time was healed when the water was stirred, the man seemed discouraged by the fact that someone else was healed before he could get to the water. Perhaps he had nearly given up hope that he would ever be healed. Perhaps Christ's question to him regenerated this man's faith. Maybe he thought Christ was volunteering to assist him the next time the water was stirred. In any case, the man wanted to be healed.

- _Jesus said to him, "Arise, take up your pallet, and walk." And immediately the man became well, and took up his pallet and began to walk._

Christ commanded the man to get up, pick up the pallet upon which he was lying and to walk. The fact that Christ commanded him to pick up his pallet meant that he was not going to be sick and lying there any longer. The man became well immediately after Christ commanded him to arise, and he picked up his pallet and began to walk.

- *Now it was the Sabbath on that day...*

John draws the reader's attention to the fact that this healing occurred on the Sabbath. This man got into considerable trouble with those who saw him carrying his pallet. These religious critics felt he was violating the Sabbath prohibition of working.

When his critics asked who healed him, the man did not know it was Christ. *This is extremely encouraging.* Christ apparently healed a man that had not expressed faith in Him in any way that has been previously seen. Sometimes people are healed that do not seem to meet the normal conditions of faith for healing. In fact, it often seems that a kind of *hopeful neutrality* may receive healing if the person praying for them *believes.* However, the *unbelief* of a possible recipient of healing seems to *neutralize the faith* of the person praying for them. Occasionally, Christ was limited in how much He could help by the unbelief of people.

Christ met this man in the temple after his healing and warned him of potential future problems if his behavior did not change.

- *Afterward Jesus found him in the temple, and said to him, "Behold, you have become well; do not sin anymore, so that nothing worse may befall you."*

The words of Christ to the healed man in the temple seem much like a *warning* to him. Christ warned him that if he continued in sin something worse could happen to him. Since the man had been sick for thirty-eight years, it is hard to imagine what might be worse. This would be true except that Christ might be referring to the eternal consequences of unforgiven sin. However, since Christ tells the man he is well, and connects this with the warning about sin, it is likely that Christ was telling him he could get sick again if he continued sinning. There is no indication what particular sin Christ could be addressing, or if He was speaking only in a general sense. The fact that Christ does not address this man's need for forgiveness also suggests that when he was healed, that he started fresh with the Father in the matter of sin.

It is not entirely clear if Christ was telling him that his sin caused his sickness to begin with. Clearly, some sins can result in long-term illness. For instance, a sexual sin can result in an infection that could last a lifetime. Likewise, sinful abuses of alcohol will eventually produce sickness in a person. However, many other sins do not always seem to have an obvious long-term effect on the health of a person. Thankfully, despite the cause of a sickness, the Father is willing to forgive and heal through Christ.

Performing Miracles and Healing

If Christ was trying to connect this man's sins with his condition, he did not seem to address the problem in the beginning. Christ said nothing to the man about a need to repent or to be forgiven before his healing. In fact, some time had transpired before Christ said anything to him about sin at all. It seems much more likely that Christ was warning him about the potential for him to lose his healing and get sick again if he continued in sin.

Some have pointed out that not everyone who was sick was healed at this pool except this man. To some who are trying to substantiate that it is not the Father's will to heal everyone this seems like proof. However, this is a misunderstanding of Christ's ministry. Christ did not heal every sick person in every city that He ministered in. In fact, in those passages which say that He *healed all*, it is clear that the texts are referring to healing *all who came to Him*. Those who came for healing were demonstrating some expectation, some faith. Those who did not come were demonstrating that they did not believe He could help them. To be sure, there were also those who simply did not hear about Him and were not healed.

In this incident by the pool at Bethesda, these people did not come to the pool to be healed by Christ. They had come to be healed in another way. This incident is unlike those situations where Christ healed great numbers of people. In those situations, the people responded in faith to Christ and came in multitudes. In this incident, there is no faith in Christ being demonstrated openly by anyone. The people at this pool are either unaware that Christ is near or simply do not believe. It is unfortunate that some try to build a case from this incident that it must be God's will for some to remain sick since Christ did not heal everyone here. It is unfortunate that these obvious differences in conditions are overlooked.

Christ ability to heal the sick was governed by faith in a positive and negative sense. The example of what happened in Nazareth illustrates this clearly. Christ had capacity to help people in many other parts of Palestine. However, in His own hometown, He was limited in His ability to heal, deliver and do miracles because their unbelief.

The Faith of Friends Brings Healing

The next story is encouraging in some of the same ways that the story of the healing of the man at the pool of Bethesda. The time of this miracle was very early in Christ's ministry, before Christ had gathered all of His twelve disciples. The setting was a home in Galilee. Here is the first half of the story:

> *And it came about one day that He was teaching; and there were some Pharisees and teachers of the law sitting there, who had come from every village of Galilee and Judea and from Jerusalem; and the power of the Lord was present for Him to perform healing. And behold, some men were carrying on a bed a man who was paralyzed; and they were trying to bring him in, and to set him down in front of Him. And not finding any way to bring him in because of the crowd, they went up on the roof and let him*

down through the tiles with his stretcher, right in the center, in front of Jesus. Luke 5:17-19

The first half of this story sets the stage for an important healing miracle that offers some encouraging information about faith for healing. The story begins with letting the reader know that the audience for Christ's teaching in this case was very mixed and contained some potential critics.

- *And it came about one day that He was teaching; and there were some Pharisees and teachers of the law sitting there, who had come from every village of Galilee and Judea and from Jerusalem...*

Christ's fame had spread abroad, and some had made journey's to hear Christ teach and, obviously, to see His miracles and healing. The passage does not reveal exactly what Christ was teaching, but it does reveal some specifics about healing.

- *...and the power of the Lord was present for Him to perform healing.*

This story occurs very early in Luke's Gospel. In fact, before this occasion, Luke records only one *mass* healing event, two healings of individuals and one individual delivered from demons. The Scripture statement above is unusual, and it seems to imply that some *special* manifestation of the power of the Lord is necessary to heal the sick. However, when a survey is taken throughout the New Testament concerning Christ's healing ministry to the masses, there are *no other statements* like it. Perhaps Luke wanted to particularly emphasize that Christ was dependent upon the power of the Holy Spirit in healing ministry or that there was an *unusually strong presence* of the Holy Spirit healing the multitude through Christ on this occasion. On occasion, in modern healing meetings, as faith arises in a congregation, an unusually strong presence of the power of the Holy Spirit may come and greater miracles may be the result. However, much healing can be accomplished *without an unusual presence* of the Holy Spirit. Since there were many critics present, perhaps Luke is telling his readers that the Holy Spirit came with unusually great power and presence to reveal Christ as Healer on this occasion.

- *And behold, some men were carrying on a bed a man who was paralyzed; and they were trying to bring him in, and to set him down in front of Him. And not finding any way to bring him in because of the crowd, they went up on the roof and let him down through the tiles with his stretcher, right in the center, in front of Jesus.*

The story continues with the details of these men trying to bring this paralyzed man to Christ for healing. The large crowd in the house, and apparently outside as well, seemed to block them from entering the house with the paralyzed man on his stretcher. However, this was not enough difficulty to stop these men. They instead went up on the roof, removed some tiles and boldly lowered the man so that he was lying right in front of Christ. There must have been a few moments where Christ stopped His ministry to see what they were doing with this man. The second half of this story now follows:

> _And seeing their faith, He said, "Friend, your sins are forgiven you." And the scribes and the Pharisees began to reason, saying, "Who is this man who speaks blasphemies? Who can forgive sins, but God alone?" But Jesus, aware of their reasonings, answered and said to them, "Why are you reasoning in your hearts? Which is easier, to say, 'Your sins have been forgiven you,' or to say, 'Rise and walk'? But in order that you may know that the Son of Man has authority on earth to forgive sins,"-- He said to the paralytic-- "I say to you, rise, and take up your stretcher and go home." And he took up what he had been lying on, and went home, glorifying God. And they were all seized with astonishment and began glorifying God; and they were filled with fear, saying, "We have seen remarkable things today." Luke 5:20-26_

Christ saw _their faith_. In other words, the faith of the friends of this man is what is noteworthy. The friends of this man were still on the housetop but _their faith_ revealed in their boldness and persistence on behalf of their friend is what Christ noticed.

- _And seeing their faith, He said, "Friend, your sins are forgiven you."_

While Christ noticed the faith of the men on the housetop, the _beneficiary_ of _their faith_ was the paralyzed man lying in front of Christ. This is extremely encouraging. The faith of friends and family can release blessing to others perhaps that are not believing for themselves. Perhaps that is what happened to the sick man at Bethesda's Pool. Perhaps he had friends or family that believed for him. However, this is pure speculation, as the text gives no specific evidence of this. Because of his friends' faith, Christ said to this paralyzed man that his sins were forgiven. This statement drew the ire of the religious critics present.

- _And the scribes and the Pharisees began to reason, saying, "Who is this man who speaks blasphemies? Who can forgive sins, but God alone?"_

The logic of Christ's critics is clear. Christ has just forgiven this man his sins. Since God alone can forgive sins, Christ is taking upon Himself a role that God alone assumes. This would be _blasphemy_ if Christ were not God. However, since Christ is God the Son, He was speaking the truth. However, there must be something more here that may not be entirely evident. Christ's reaction to His critics reveals important information about spiritual authority and the connection between healing and forgiveness.

- _But Jesus, aware of their reasonings, answered and said to them, "Why are you reasoning in your hearts? Which is easier, to say, 'Your sins have been forgiven you,' or to say, 'Rise and walk'?"_

Performing Miracles and Healing

The problem with these religious critics was their _reasonings_ about Christ. This is the problem today as well, people often wrongly reason about healing and come to unbelieving conclusions. This is because they simply do not fully know the Scriptures and have not experienced the magnitude of the power of God.

In this man's case, Christ makes an important connection between forgiveness of sins and healing. Christ is saying to His critics that _when someone receives healing isn't the Father demonstrating His forgiveness of them as well?_ Since Christ was revealing the Father in all matters, Christ's mercy in healing these people reveals more than just the Father's willingness to heal. Healing them reveals the Father's forgiveness of all their sins as well. The critics of Christ, however, were focused on His taking the role of the Father in forgiving sins. Christ knew before He said this that the critics would react. Christ was not bound by the fear of man or by false humility. He took the occasion to shock them with the truth despite their potentially negative reaction. Christ then demonstrated to His critics that He had authority to forgive sins on earth by healing the man.

- _But in order that you may know that the Son of Man has authority on earth to forgive sins,"-- He said to the paralytic-- "I say to you, rise, and take up your stretcher and go home." and he took up what he had been lying on, and went home, glorifying God._

The truth of a teaching or a doctrine is evaluated partly by the Holy Spirit's willingness to attest to its truth by changing people's lives. In other words, Christ demonstrated what He had said about forgiveness. The Holy Spirit attested to the fact that invisible forgiveness was being received by doing visible healings.

Christ said that He was the *Son of Man* rather than the *Son of God* in this passage. While Christ is both, the emphasis here is upon His role as the *Anointed One*. The term *Son of Man* is generally accepted to be a messianic title found in the Old Testament. However, Christ's use of this title rather than emphasis on the fact that He was divine Himself, indicates that Christ was operating as a man rather than as God. In fact, Christ said that He had *authority on earth* to forgive sins. This suggests that the Father had given Him authority rather than Him having authority simply because He was God.

Likewise, believers have authority to offer forgiveness of sins. This does not mean that believers can offer forgiveness without conditions of repentance or faith. Even Christ did not have authority to forgive sins without the proper conditions. Believers stand in Christ's authority releasing people by inspiration of the Holy Spirit into all of Christ's provision for them in matters of guilt and shame. They become active agents of forgiveness, confirming, encouraging and boldly releasing people into the mercy of God provided at the cross of Christ. Therefore, the two matters of healing and forgiveness of sin are so intimately connected that when they are disconnected, nothing will work quite right in ministry.

Performing Miracles and Healing

There is a great need in our day for Christian people to be confirmed in their forgiveness, to be released from shame, and to be given permission to do the works of Christ despite their failures. Many people await permission to do those things that Christ has already told them to do. Failures and sins produce the feelings of not having any real authority and of needing permission. Anyone seeking to heal the sick and to equip others to do so will find himself or herself continually dealing with guilt and shame in people, and thereby authorizing them to be bold in Christ.

The story ends with the reaction of the people to this healing. Christ had apparently made His point with His critics. The wording of the reactions of the people here, including the critics is particularly strong.

- *And they were all seized with astonishment and began glorifying God; and they were filled with fear, saying, "We have seen remarkable things today."*

They were *seized*. They were *astonished*. They *glorified God*. They were *filled with fear*. They had seen *remarkable things* that day. The strongly expressive language indicates that this was an unusual set of events. As indicated earlier in the discussion that there might have been an unusual presence of God in this setting that distinguished it from many other times when Christ healed the sick.

The Man with Dropsy

The story of the man with dropsy has some points of interest. No one is exactly sure what *dropsy* is. The Greek word translated *dropsy* is only used in this passage. It is the Greek word *hydropikos*. The first part of the word is familiar. The Greek word *hydro* means *water*. Some have suggested that *dropsy* is *edema*, a severe swelling caused by excessive water in the tissues or even a possible tumor. However, no one seems to know for sure and modern versions often use the King James word *dropsy* for lack of a modern term. This story is also interesting because it emphasizes a particular illustration that Christ draws about healing. Here is the story found only in Luke's Gospel.

> *And it came about when He went into the house of one of the leaders of the Pharisees on the Sabbath to eat bread, that they were watching Him closely. And there, in front of Him was a certain man suffering from dropsy. And Jesus answered and spoke to the lawyers and Pharisees, saying, " Is it lawful to heal on the Sabbath, or not? " But they kept silent. And He took hold of him, and healed him, and sent him away. And He said to them, "Which one of you shall have a son or an ox fall into a well, and will not immediately pull him out on a Sabbath day?" And they could make no reply to this. Luke 14:1-6*

This story starts with Christ entering the home of a potential critic to eat a meal. Christ obviously was not afraid of criticism. Those that were present were watching him closely to find fault.

- *And it came about when He went into the house of one of the leaders of the Pharisees on the Sabbath to eat bread, that they were watching Him closely. And there, in front of Him was a certain man suffering from dropsy. And Jesus answered and spoke to the lawyers and Pharisees, saying, " Is it lawful to heal on the Sabbath, or not?" But they kept silent.*

The passage does not reveal who this man was or why he was inside the house. He could have been a family member of one of the Pharisees or lawyers present. However, since Christ sent the man away after healing him this is unlikely. This situation could have been set up as a trap for Christ. Perhaps the critics wanted Christ to encounter this man and heal him on the Sabbath so that they could criticize. Christ possibly knowing this asks the direct question to them. *Is it lawful to heal on the Sabbath or not?* The question reveals a hidden accusation of the critics. This is the hidden accusation: *If Christ is violating the Law of Moses when He heals, then God must not be doing the healing.* The same sort of accusation exists today in this form: *If God is not healing today, then those that are healing must be healing by some other power than God.* Christ did not yield in fear of His critics, in fact after asking the question, He answered it strongly by healing the man.

- *And He took hold of him, and healed him, and sent him away.*

Then Christ offered a powerful illustration to His critics of the relationship of healing to normal compassion.

- *And He said to them, "Which one of you shall have a son or an ox fall into a well, and will not immediately pull him out on a Sabbath day?" And they could make no reply to this.*

Normal compassion and reasonable care is not a violation of the Law on any day including the Sabbath. Christ said that healing is like the care that one would exercise if their son had fallen into a well or the compassion that would be exercised to help a domestic animal fallen into a well.   In other words, Christ is presenting sickness as *falling into a well* and healing as the *normal care and compassion* of someone helping them out of the well. This is completely consistent with what Christ reveals about the Law in other passages. Christ reveals that all the Law and the commandments are summed up in the two greatest commandments; *to love God with all your heart, mind, soul and strength and to love your neighbor as yourself.* In this case, healing someone does not violate the intent of the Law of Moses' Sabbath prohibitions since God's ultimate purpose in giving the Law was love. Showing genuine love is *always* lawful.

Man with a Withered Hand
The healing of the man with the withered hand has some similar aspects as the healing of the man with dropsy. For instance, Christ's critics are present again looking for a reason to accuse Him. This is another time when Christ

healed someone on the Sabbath in front of His critics. This story is found in all the Gospels except the Gospel of John. Here is the story from Luke's Gospel:

> *And He was saying to them, "The Son of Man is Lord of the Sabbath." And it came about on another Sabbath, that He entered the synagogue and was teaching; and there was a man there whose right hand was withered. And the scribes and the Pharisees were watching Him closely, to see if He healed on the Sabbath, in order that they might find reason to accuse Him. But He knew what they were thinking, and He said to the man with the withered hand, "Rise and come forward!" And he rose and came forward. And Jesus said to them, "I ask you, is it lawful on the Sabbath to do good, or to do harm, to save a life, or to destroy it?" And after looking around at them all, He said to him, "Stretch out your hand!" And he did so; and his hand was restored. But they themselves were filled with rage, and discussed together what they might do to Jesus. Luke 6:5-11*

The story begins with Christ stating that He is Lord of the Sabbath. This statement comes right after a controversy with His critics about the disciples feeding themselves by rubbing heads of wheat in their hands to remove the hull. The Pharisees thought that the disciples were violating the Sabbath work prohibition by feeding themselves in this manner. Christ reminds them of a biblical hero, King David, doing something that was similar. Christ then tells them that He is Lord of the Sabbath.

- *And He was saying to them, "The Son of Man is Lord of the Sabbath."*

This bold statement to His critics simply meant that He was the rightful judge of what violated the Sabbath and not his critics. Since Christ represented the Father's word and will, He revealed the Father's kind intentions on the Sabbath as He did every other day.

- *And it came about on another Sabbath, that He entered the synagogue and was teaching; and there was a man there whose right hand was withered. And the scribes and the Pharisees were watching Him closely, to see if He healed on the Sabbath, in order that they might find reason to accuse Him.*

Luke illustrates what Christ meant by saying He was Lord of the Sabbath by immediately telling his readers what happened on *another Sabbath.* In the midst of unbelieving critics looking for a reason to accuse Him, Christ encountered a man who had a withered right hand.

- *But He knew what they were thinking, and He said to the man with the withered hand, "Rise and come forward!" And he rose and came forward.*

In spite of the fact that they were waiting to accuse Him, Christ called the man forward. The man responded to

Christ's command and came forward. Christ then asked His critics a question about the Sabbath.

- *And Jesus said to them, "I ask you, is it lawful on the Sabbath to do good, or to do harm, to save a life, or to destroy it?"*

This question reveals the accusation that Christ was violating the law of the Sabbath in a new light. Christ presents two choices. He compares healing the man with doing nothing for the man. Healing the man would be *doing good* and *saving a life*. Failure to heal the man when He could would be *doing harm* and *destroying a life*. The answer of the question is obvious. It is always lawful *to do good* and *to save a life* by *healing* someone.

- *And after looking around at them all, He said to him, "Stretch out your hand!" And he did so; and his hand was restored.*

It suggests that Christ boldly obtained eye contact with every critic and then healed this man. The man's hand was restored as the man obeyed Christ's command to stretch out his hand. Christ *fearlessly* did *good* in healing people, despite the amount of opposition.

- *But they themselves were filled with rage, and discussed together what they might do to Jesus.*

Despite the fact that Christ went about and did good and healed all that were oppressed of the devil, human opposition was almost always present. Anyone thinking that they can have a healing and miracle ministry without having opposition is going to be surprised where the opposition may come from when they regularly heal the sick. If Christ was opposed in His perfect reflection of the Father's will, then those who are less than perfect will also suffer opposition. However, Christ occasionally won over His critics. His followers should show the same patience, trusting that the Father can melt the hardest heart. Sometimes religious opposition will be found in family and Christians leaders with a differing view on healing. Anyone wishing to continue to help the suffering must stand firm on Scripture and be patient in the face of opposition.

The High Priest's Slave

The last event of healing in this chapter is the final time that Christ ministered to someone before the cross and resurrection. The injury to the slave of the High Priest is revealed in all four Gospels. However, Christ's healing of him is only mentioned in Luke's Gospel. Here is the brief story:

> _And a certain one of them struck the slave of the high priest and cut off his right ear. But Jesus answered and said, "Stop! No more of this." And He touched his ear and healed him. Luke 22:50-51_

Peter defended Christ with a sword and cut off this man's right ear. Christ put a stop to His disciples defending Him with violence and healed this man's ear. In the face of this threatening mob that had set out to take Him by force, Christ had consideration for the physical well-being of this enemy. After He healed the man, Christ was led away to be accused and eventually crucified. His crucifixion, however, purchased eternal salvation, healing and deliverance for all that will believe. His resurrection and the gift of the Holy Spirit now ensure that the Holy Spirit, working in His Church, will duplicate His ministry.

~10~

Christ Raises the Dead

The Raising of Jairus' Daughter

Scripture reveals that Christ raised three people from the dead during His earthly ministry. Since Christ commanded His disciples to also raise the dead, it is necessary to review the New Testament on this kind of supernatural ministry. Raising the dead is not exactly healing but has many similarities in the way that it is revealed in the New Testament. The story of the raising of Jairus' daughter is a good place to begin.

> *And behold, there came a man named Jairus, and he was an official of the synagogue; and he fell at Jesus' feet, and began to entreat Him to come to his house; for he had an only daughter, about twelve years old, and she was dying. But as He went, the multitudes were pressing against Him...*
> *Luke 8:41-42*

Performing Miracles and Healing

The story begins with Christ hearing the synagogue official's request for Christ to come heal his dying daughter. Christ responded positively to this request and went with Jairus. On the way to Jairus' home, the masses of people were pressing against Christ. The healing of the woman with a twelve-year issue of blood takes place next in this passage. In other words, "sandwiched" between the beginning and end of the story of the raising of Jairus' daughter from the dead, is the healing of the woman with the issue of blood. Since this healing was covered in another part of this book, it is unnecessary to review it again. Here is the continuation and end of the story of Jairus' daughter:

> *While He was still speaking (to the woman who had been healed), someone came from the house of the synagogue official, saying, "Your daughter has died; do not trouble the Teacher anymore." But when Jesus heard this, He answered him, "Do not be afraid any longer; only believe, and she shall be made well." And when He had come to the house, He did not allow anyone to enter with Him, except Peter and John and James, and the girl's father and mother. Now they were all weeping and lamenting for her; but He said, "Stop weeping, for she has not died, but is asleep." And they began laughing at Him, knowing that she had died. He, however, took her by the hand and called, saying, "Child, arise!" And her spirit returned, and she rose immediately; and He gave orders for something to be given her to eat. And her parents were amazed; but He instructed them to tell no one what had happened. Luke 8:49-56*

Christ Raises the Dead

The story reveals that Christ was informed of the change in status of Jairus' daughter on the way to heal her. Someone from Jairus' house came to give him the bad news.

- *While He was still speaking (to the woman who had been healed), someone came from the house of the synagogue official, saying, "Your daughter has died; do not trouble the Teacher anymore."*

Many who believe in healing today would assume that the opportunity had passed for God to be glorified in this situation. However, Christ did not react this way. It is clear that Christ believed what He had taught, specifically that all things were possible to the person who believes.

- *But when Jesus heard this, He answered him, "Do not be afraid any longer; only believe, and she shall be made well."*

Jairus' reaction is very normal for the circumstance, he is *afraid* that his ill daughter is now dead. While there is evidence of faith in Jairus seeking out Christ for help, the circumstance had gotten worse since he encountered Christ. Any parent facing the reality of a dying child would naturally be afraid. When Jairus received a reliable report that his daughter was dead, *fear* overtook him. However, Christ revealed that Jairus' *believing* would be the key for his daughter *to be made well*.

This story should encourage parents facing a serious condition affecting their child. First, it seems that Christ looked to Jairus, as the parent, to believe. Secondly, Christ encouraged Jairus not to *fear* any longer. Fear and faith seem to be opposites in many passages in Scripture. Fear believes that something bad can happen. True faith in Christ, however, believes that something good will happen.

This is often where complex theology causes problems in people's faith by trying to convince believers that something bad is actually a mysterious good. This kind of theological confusion makes it difficult not to fear and difficult to have a clear faith to receive the Father's answer.

Often because of tragedies of the past, there is fear in many ministers facing a serious potentially fatal condition in a child. These ministers sometimes have adopted a theology that will preempt and weaken the possibility of a miracle. Often the real reason that these ministers have adopted unbelieving theologies, is that they are afraid to face situations where a child might be dying. These ministers can come and prepare the family for the death of a child and have the appearance of wisdom. These ministers may be actually protecting themselves from the criticism of failure to heal the child.

While a person lives there is possibility for healing. Even after a person has died, there is possibility for a short season for a resurrection and a healing. After all, what is impossible normally is certainly possible for God. A God that heals colds, can certainly heal cancer. A God who will remove a wart, certainly will remove a tumor. A God who can heal cancer, certainly can raise a dead person. Nothing is impossible for him who believes.

There is great confusion in our day between true faith and many other similar but different things. Faith is not trust. Faith is not sincerity. Faith is not hope. Faith is not desperation. Faith is not compassion or great desire. Faith is not perseverance in prayer. While faith may be mixed with some of these other good things, it is not any of these things. Faith simply believes in the reliability of God. Faith is the soul actively positioned on the reliability of the Father to save, heal and deliver in a specific matter. Faith is the substance of things hoped for and the evidence of things not yet seen. True faith always obtains those specific things that are the good intentions of the Father. True faith fights through fear and receives the good intentions of the Father.

- *And when He had come to the house, He did not allow anyone to enter with Him, except Peter and John and James, and the girl's father and mother.*

When Christ arrived, He purposely limited the number of people that were present in the house where the dead girl was. There were five people present with Christ, including the parents of the girl. Christ had told the father earlier, *"only believe, and she shall be made well."* In other words, the father's faith was important to this resurrection. Since Christ had already acknowledged that faith was important, it is rather certain that His limiting the number of people present in the room had to do with faith.

- _Now they were all weeping and lamenting for her; but He said, "Stop weeping, for she has not died, but is asleep." And they began laughing at Him, knowing that she had died._

It appears that the people Christ had taken in the house where the daughter was were laughing at Christ. However, when the three parallel accounts[1] of this story are studied, it is clear that this is a description of the _crowds_ reaction _before_ Christ went in the house. The crowd laughed at what Christ said about the girl's condition. In other words, they could not believe even for a second that their diagnosis of the finality of this situation could be wrong. Christ allowed none of these unbelieving people into the house. Christ carefully controlled the conditions of this miracle. Only three of His disciples and the parents of the girl were allowed inside.

- _He, however, took her by the hand and called, saying, "Child, arise!" And her spirit returned, and she rose immediately; and He gave orders for something to be given her to eat._

Christ simply spoke to the girl commanding her to do what would be normal for a healing. Christ simply told her to get up. The passage says that her _spirit returned_. The word _spirit_ is translated from the Greek word _pnema_. This Greek word can be alternatively translated as _breath_ or _wind_. A substitution of the word _breath_ for _spirit_ here would make some sense. The passage then would say _And_

---

[1] The three accounts of this resurrection are found in Matthew 9:18-26, Mark 5:21-43, and Luke 8:40-56

her breath returned. In other words, the girl began to breathe again. This was probably how they knew she had died. She had quit breathing. In addition, while the passage does not say so, a good assumption would be that the girl got up healed from whatever had caused her death.

- *And her parents were amazed...*

It is clear that the girl had died. No one would be *amazed* otherwise. The account does not reveal how long exactly she had been dead. However, it does appear that she had been dead only a short time. Another resurrection in Christ's ministry occurred after the man was dead for four days and already buried. There seems to be no clear rules in the matter of resurrections from the dead. While there seems to be no evidence of specific guidance by the Holy Spirit in the matter of the resurrection of Jairus' daughter, there does seem to be some indication of specific guidance in the resurrection of Lazarus.

The Resurrection of Lazarus

Scripture provides a detailed account of the matters surrounding the resurrection of Lazarus. In fact, there is so much important detail that the long passage requires some divisions in order to deal with it intelligently. Therefore, here is the first of five parts of this passage.

> *Now a certain man was sick, Lazarus of Bethany, the village of Mary and her sister Martha... The sisters therefore sent to Him, saying, "Lord, behold, he whom You love is sick." But when Jesus heard it, He said, "This sickness is not unto death, but for the*

glory of God, that the Son of God may be glorified by it." Now Jesus loved Martha, and her sister, and Lazarus. When therefore He heard that he was sick, He stayed then two days longer in the place where He was. Then after this He said to the disciples, "Let us go to Judea again." John 11:1, 3-7

The passage begins by introducing details about a particular family that lived in the village of Bethany. The account reveals that this family had a strikingly intimate relationship with Christ.

- *Now a certain man was sick, Lazarus of Bethany, the village of Mary and her sister Martha... The sisters therefore sent to Him, saying, "Lord, behold, he whom You love is sick."*

It is obvious that Christ was a friend with this family. The sisters even identified their brother as *he whom You love* rather than naming Lazarus. Christ's reaction to this situation was somewhat different. Normally, Christ immediately responded to information like this and healed the person involved. Christ did not seem to need divine guidance to respond in that fashion. In contrast, Christ appeared to have some specific revelation about this situation that He was obeying.

- *But when Jesus heard it, He said, "This sickness is not unto death, but for the glory of God, that the Son of God may be glorified by it."*

Christ Raises the Dead

Christ seemed to know that this situation was unusual and different from His normal ministry to the sick. Christ knew that the sickness was not to cause Lazarus' death at this time. Since Lazarus did die, it would be interesting to know exactly what Christ did know and when He knew it. Most likely, Christ knew only in part and obtained additional guidance from the Father as the situation progressed. There is evidence in the passage to indicate that Christ did not know all the details of this situation in advance. A careful reading of the passage does not support the alternative, that Christ knew every detail in advance. The passage does support that He knew some important things in advance.

There has been some confusion in the minds of some about what glorified God in this circumstance. Is Lazarus' sickness or death what brought God glory? *No!* If Lazarus had remained sick or had just died, then God would not have been glorified at all. Christ revealing Himself as the one who raises from the dead was what brought glory to God. Lazarus' resurrection and healing from the sickness that caused his death is what brought God the glory. If Lazarus had simply died, it is unlikely that the story of his sickness and death would be in the Bible at all, because it would not have revealed Christ or glorified the Father.

- *Now Jesus loved Martha, and her sister, and Lazarus. When therefore He heard that he was sick, He stayed then two days longer in the place where He was. Then after this He said to the disciples, "Let us go to Judea again."*

Instead of Christ immediately responding to this situation as He normally did, He showed some more signs of specific Divine guidance in this matter. Christ stayed *two more days* where He was before leaving for Bethany with His disciples. In other words, Christ purposely delayed His arriving where His sick friend Lazarus was. Since, when He actually arrived, Lazarus had been dead for more than four days, clearly Lazarus would have been dead before Christ could have arrived even if He left immediately. The Father's purpose in delaying Christ must have been to create a greater miracle of resurrection. Instead of Lazarus being dead two days, he was dead for more than four days and had begun to decay. Here is part two of the five parts of this story:

> *This He said, and after that He said to them, "Our friend Lazarus has fallen asleep; but I go, that I may awaken him out of sleep." The disciples therefore said to Him, "Lord, if he has fallen asleep, he will recover." Now Jesus had spoken of his death, but they thought that He was speaking of literal sleep. Then Jesus therefore said to them plainly, "Lazarus is dead, and I am glad for your sakes that I was not there, so that you may believe; but let us go to him."...So when Jesus came, He found that he had already been in the tomb four days. John 11:11-15, 17*

Christ used some familiar figurative language as He addressed Lazarus' condition. Christ spoke of *death* being *sleep*. In the resurrection account of Jairus' daughter, Christ told the crowd that the dead girl was *sleeping*. In fact,

Christ Raises the Dead

Christ did nothing more than the actions someone would take in *awakening* someone from *sleep*. He simply spoke to her and took her hand. Christ used the same metaphor in this account. He told the disciples that He was going to *awaken Lazarus from sleep.*

- *This He said, and after that He said to them, "Our friend Lazarus has fallen asleep; but I go, that I may awaken him out of sleep." The disciples therefore said to Him, "Lord, if he has fallen asleep, he will recover." Now Jesus had spoken of his death, but they thought that He was speaking of literal sleep.*

This is the first time that the disciples have understood clearly what has happened to Lazarus.

- *Then Jesus therefore said to them plainly, "Lazarus is dead, and I am glad for your sakes that I was not there, so that you may believe; but let us go to him."...So when Jesus came, He found that he had already been in the tomb four days.*

Christ revealed that the disciples should have their faith strengthened by these events. For one thing, Christ knew supernaturally that Lazarus had died. If Christ had been there when Lazarus had died then this would have not revealed anything about Christ. However, the disciples ought to have had their faith strengthened because of Christ's prior knowledge of these events.

When Christ and His disciples arrived, they discovered that Lazarus had been dead more than four days. In other words, Christ did not know exactly what the situation was. He did not know exactly how long Lazarus had been dead. This is evidence that Christ knew only in part.

After arriving at Bethany, Christ encountered one of the grieving sisters. Here is the third part of the five parts of this continuing story:

> *Martha therefore, when she heard that Jesus was coming, went to meet Him; but Mary still sat in the house. Martha therefore said to Jesus, "Lord, if You had been here, my brother would not have died. "Even now I know that whatever You ask of God, God will give You." Jesus said to her, "Your brother shall rise again." Martha said to Him, "I know that he will rise again in the resurrection on the last day." Jesus said to her, "I am the resurrection and the life; he who believes in Me shall live even if he dies, and everyone who lives and believes in Me shall never die. Do you believe this? " She said to Him, "Yes, Lord; I have believed that You are the Christ, the Son of God, even He who comes into the world." John 11:20-27*

Martha was very much aware of Christ's capacity to heal the sick. She immediately reacted to Christ's presence with that thought in her mind.

- *Martha therefore said to Jesus, "Lord, if You had been here, my brother would not have died. "Even now I*

*know that whatever You ask of God, God will give
You."*

Martha also knew that a possibility existed of
Lazarus' resurrection. This story occurred just before
Christ entered Jerusalem during the last week of His life.
Christ had accomplished two other resurrections before
these events. Christ had raised Jairus' daughter and the
widow's son from the dead. Martha was surely aware of
those events but unsure about what Christ would do with
her brother Lazarus. Martha seemed to know that the
Father would give Christ whatever He asked. She was not
asking *if Christ could* raise Lazarus from the dead. She
knew that Christ could do it. Her implicit but silent
question was *will you raise my brother from the dead?*
Christ answered her unstated question very directly. He
said that He would raise Lazarus from the dead.

- *Jesus said to her, "Your brother shall rise again."
  Martha said to Him, "I know that he will rise again in
  the resurrection on the last day."*

Martha obviously understood that any resurrection
in Christ's earthly ministry is temporary. The person will
have to die again. And she understood the resurrection to
come that is eternal. She was asking for clarification from
Christ. She knew that Christ would raise Lazarus eternally
in the future. Did Christ mean that Lazarus was going to be
raised up *eternally* or *temporarily*? What she really desired
was Lazarus' temporary resurrection then. Christ's answer
to her was revealing.

- *Jesus said to her, "I am the resurrection and the life; he who believes in Me shall live even if he dies, and everyone who lives and believes in Me shall never die. Do you believe this?"*

Christ encouraged her to *believe* in Him. Christ did not answer her question directly but solicited a faith response from her. Three times in these few words, Christ said something about *believing* in Him or asked her if she *believed*. Martha then answered Christ's question.

- *She said to Him, "Yes, Lord; I have believed that You are the Christ, the Son of God, even He who comes into the world."*

A powerful believing response flowed from Martha's heart. She had a clear revelation of who Christ was, despite her grief over the loss of her brother. Christ had not answered her implicit question about her brother but she believed in Christ. She did not understand entirely what might happen, but she believed in Christ. The fourth part of this five-part story now introduces Martha's sister to the situation.

Therefore, when Mary came where Jesus was, she saw Him, and fell at His feet, saying to Him, "Lord, if You had been here, my brother would not have died." When Jesus therefore saw her (Mary) weeping, and the Jews who came with her, also weeping, He was deeply moved in spirit, and was troubled, and said, "Where have you laid him?" They said to Him, "Lord, come and see." Jesus wept. And so the Jews were saying, "Behold how He loved him!" But some of them said, "Could not this man, who opened the eyes of him who was blind, have kept this man also from dying?" John 11:32-37

Mary reacted in similar fashion, as did Martha when she first encountered Christ. Mary was aware that Christ could have healed Lazarus if He had been present.

- *Therefore, when Mary came where Jesus was, she saw Him, and fell at His feet, saying to Him, "Lord, if You had been here, my brother would not have died."*

The account does not give a specific discourse between Christ and Mary as it did between Christ and Martha. However, Christ reacted strongly to Mary's pain of loss, as well as to those who were actually grieving over the loss of Lazarus.

- *When Jesus therefore saw her (Mary) weeping, and the Jews who came with her, also weeping, He was deeply moved in spirit, and was troubled, and said, "Where have you laid him?" They said to Him, "Lord, come and see." Jesus wept. And so the Jews were saying, "Behold how He loved him!"*

Christ's emotion in these verses is apparent. He was *deeply moved in spirit, troubled* and even *wept*. However, exactly what Christ was feeling is not entirely apparent. It strongly appears that He was experiencing normal grief Himself, perhaps just as a reaction to the emotional pain of the people around Him. In other passages, sometimes they relate that Christ, *moved with compassion, healed the sick.*

• *But some of them said, "Could not this man, who opened the eyes of him who was blind, have kept this man also from dying?"*

Those who were present were aware of the capacity of Christ to heal the sick, the injured and the disabled. They referred to Christ's capacity to heal the blind as a focal point. In other words, their logic was good if not limited. They understood that if a man could heal the blind, then why should anything be difficult beyond that? Actually, the blind are not harder to heal than a common cold. Since it is not the believer who actually heals but Christ, then one healing or miracle is actually no more difficult than another. There is a kind of divine paradox present. The believer must simply believe that one thing is no harder than another. They must know that they are not actually doing it although they are being *used* to do it.

This is the final or fifth part of the five parts of this story:

Jesus therefore again being deeply moved within, came to the tomb. Now it was a cave, and a stone was lying against it. Jesus said, "Remove the stone." Martha, the sister of the deceased, said to Him, "Lord, by this time there will be a stench, for he has been dead four days." Jesus said to her, "Did I not say to you, if you believe, you will see the glory of God?" And so they removed the stone. And Jesus raised His eyes, and said, "Father, I thank Thee that Thou hearest Me. And I knew that Thou hearest Me always; but because of the people standing around I said it, that they may believe that Thou didst send Me." And when He had said these things, He cried out with a loud voice, "Lazarus, come forth." He who had died came forth, bound hand and foot with wrappings; and his face was wrapped around with a cloth. Jesus said to them, "Unbind him, and let him go." Many therefore of the Jews, who had come to Mary and beheld what He had done, believed in Him. But some of them went away to the Pharisees, and told them the things which Jesus had done. John 11:38-46

The account reveals that Christ being *deeply moved within* came to the tomb. The possibility that Christ was receiving divine guidance in this matter is strongly suggested by these words. The tomb where Lazarus' body has been laid was a cave with a large stone for a door.

- *Jesus therefore again being deeply moved within, came to the tomb. Now it was a cave, and a stone was lying against it. Jesus said, "Remove the stone."*

Christ commanded that the stone be removed and got an immediate reaction from Martha. Martha suggested that removing the stone was inappropriate because the body of Lazarus would have decayed and would have produced a bad odor.

- *Martha, the sister of the deceased, said to Him, "Lord, by this time there will be a stench, for he has been dead four days."*

Martha reminded Christ that Lazarus had been dead for four days. However, Christ reminded Martha of their previous discussion about her believing in Him. He had said something repeatedly about believing in Him, and she had confessed that she did believe in Christ.

- *Jesus said to her, "Did I not say to you, if you believe, you will see the glory of God?"*

This question revealed that Martha's faith in Christ would be a condition of her seeing the glory of God. Earlier Christ had answered her implicit question about raising her brother from the dead by asking her if she believed that He was the resurrection. She had answered in the affirmative. Here Christ reminded Martha that she needed to *believe* in order to *see* the glory of God. Apparently, Martha's faith was necessary for Lazarus' resurrection to take place. While she still did not understand entirely, apparently she did believe. After they removed the stone, Christ turned His attention to the Father in an open prayer.

- *And so they removed the stone. And Jesus raised His eyes, and said, "Father, I thank Thee that Thou hearest Me. And I knew that Thou hearest Me always; but because of the people standing around I said it, that they may believe that Thou didst send Me."*

Christ Raises the Dead

Christ did not bow His head in prayer but lifted His eyes to the Father. He prayed openly so that all could hear His interaction with the Father. He even explained in His prayer that He wanted the people to know that His Father always heard Him so that they would believe that the Father had sent Him. Of course, since the first chapter, this book has emphasized that *believing* that *the Father sent Christ* is the foundation of supernatural ministry. Here Christ revealed that the raising of Lazarus was for that purpose.

- *And when He had said these things, He cried out with a loud voice, "Lazarus, come forth." He who had died came forth, bound hand and foot with wrappings; and his face was wrapped around with a cloth.*

In a manner much like someone trying to *awaken someone else* who is a distance away from them, Christ loudly commanded Lazarus to *come forth*. Lazarus then came forth all wrapped up in his shroud and grave cloths, requiring assistance to get unwrapped.

- *Jesus said to them, "Unbind him, and let him go." Many therefore of the Jews, who had come to Mary and beheld what He had done, believed in Him.*

The reaction of the people to this miracle of resurrection was precisely what Christ had intended. Those that saw the miracle believed, or they reacted as some do today. They went to Christ's enemies to report on Him.

• *But some of them went away to the Pharisees, and told them the things which Jesus had done.*

The fact of religious opposition to Christ's healing and miracle ministry is apparent then and now. The same critical, unbelieving, pharisaical spirit is with us today. Some will react to Christ's servants in these same ways as they demonstrate His works.

The Resurrection of the Widow's Son

The last resurrection account that we will review in this chapter is the resurrection of the widow's son. It is found only in Luke's Gospel, and is chronologically very early in the ministry of Christ.

Now as He approached the gate of the city (Nain), behold, a dead man was being carried out, the only son of his mother, and she was a widow; and a sizeable crowd from the city was with her. And when the Lord saw her, He felt compassion for her, and said to her, "Do not weep." And He came up and touched the coffin; and the bearers came to a halt. And He said, "Young man, I say to you, arise!" And the dead man sat up, and began to speak. And Jesus gave him back to his mother. And fear gripped them all, and they began glorifying God, saying, " A great prophet has arisen among us!" and, "God has visited His people!" And this report concerning Him went out all over Judea, and in all the surrounding district. Luke 7:12-17

Christ Raises the Dead

This resurrection is found just after the healing of the Centurion's slave. It lacks the kind of evidence of divine guidance that the resurrection in John's Gospel has. This event seems to be much more an event that happened spontaneously.

- *Now as He approached the gate of the city (Nain), behold, a dead man was being carried out, the only son of his mother, and she was a widow; and a sizeable crowd from the city was with her.*

As Christ approached the city of Nain, He encountered a sizable funeral procession. There is much detail in this short account from which to draw. The account reveals that the man who had died was the only son to a widow.

- *And when the Lord saw her, He felt compassion for her, and said to her, "Do not weep." And He came up and touched the coffin; and the bearers came to a halt.*

There does not seem to be any evidence of specific divine guidance in this account. Christ simply seemed to understand that this woman would have been without family and without help in her old age. She would have been alone, and possibly destitute. He reacted to her situation with appropriate compassion. Christ was aware that the normal course of events was for children to outlive parents. He stopped the procession by touching the coffin and again *awakening* someone who had died.

- _And He said, "Young man, I say to you, arise!" And the dead man sat up, and began to speak. And Jesus gave him back to his mother._

Christ's compassion for this woman seemed enough motivation for Him to raise her son from the dead. Again _moved with compassion_ Christ manifested the power of the Father. While faith is not specifically mentioned in this passage, certainly faith was involved. Whether Christ's personal faith or that of His disciples, or the widow, it is certain that someone or everyone believed for this miracle. Christ Himself obviously believed that He could do this, or He would not have stopped the funeral procession. This miracle produced an important effect: The people glorified God and believed in Christ.

- _And fear gripped them all, and they began glorifying God, saying, " A great prophet has arisen among us!" and, "God has visited His people!" And this report concerning Him went out all over Judea, and in all the surrounding district._

As to when a resurrection should occur in a situation, there seems to be no rules. In one situation, the death was recent, in others a number of days had passed. However, no resurrection in Scripture went for many days past the burial of the person. The longest specific amount of days revealed is four days in the case of Lazarus. In the other two accounts, the daughter of Jairus had just died and the widow's son had not yet been entombed.

Christ Raises the Dead

Obedience to the Holy Spirit, compassion for the hurting and sensitivity to the conditions for faith seem to be revealed in these accounts. While some situations seem to reveal divine guidance, others seem to be more spontaneous. Some situations apparently need to be wisely controlled where faith can flourish. Others simply need bold faith.

~11~

Two Incidents of Great Faith

The Great Faith of the Centurion

The Lord Jesus Christ praised two people and said that they had *great faith*. On both occasions, special miracles were accomplished. The Roman centurion that Christ met in Capernaum was one of these people. Here is the first part of the story found in Matthew's Gospel:

> *And when He had entered Capernaum, a centurion came to Him, entreating Him, and saying, "Lord, my servant is lying paralyzed at home, suffering great pain." And He said to him, "I will come and heal him." But the centurion answered and said, "Lord, I am not worthy for You to come under my roof, but just say the word, and my servant will be healed. "For I, too, am a man under authority, with soldiers under me; and I say to this one, 'Go!' and*

*he goes, and to another, 'Come!' and he comes, and
to my slave, 'Do this!' and he does it. "
Matthew 8:5- 9*

The first half of this story relates that a Roman
centurion, a military leader over many men, came to Jesus
Christ about his sick servant. The text says this servant was
paralyzed and in *great pain.*

- *And when He had entered Capernaum, a centurion
  came to Him, entreating Him, and saying, "Lord, my
  servant is lying paralyzed at home, suffering great
  pain." And He said to him, "I will come and heal him."*

Christ's reaction to the statement of the centurion
was immediate. He did not consider that the paralyzed or
painful condition of the centurion's servant could possibly
be the will of God. There was no will of the Father to
determine in this matter. Christ *already knew* that the
Father's will was to heal this man. Christ told the centurion
that He would come to where his servant was and heal the
servant. This was the usual pattern of Christ's ministry. He
would physically come and heal the servant perhaps by the
laying on of hands. However, the centurion had something
else in mind.

- *But the centurion answered and said, "Lord, I am not
  worthy for You to come under my roof, but just say the
  word, and my servant will be healed.*

The centurion responded to Christ with great
humility and spiritual insight. The centurion suggested an

alternative course of action. Instead of Christ coming to where the afflicted man was and laying His hands upon the servant, the centurion knew that all Christ needed to do was *speak the word* and his servant would be healed. The centurion then explained how he knew that this was possible.

- *"For I, too, am a man under authority, with soldiers under me; and I say to this one, 'Go!' and he goes, and to another, 'Come!' and he comes, and to my slave, 'Do this!' and he does it."*

The centurion said that *like Christ* he was *a man under authority.* He did not say that he was a man *in* authority. The centurion understood that *authority* is present where true *submission* is evidenced. He knew that he could verbally command soldiers under him *only* because he submitted to and obeyed the orders of his superior officer above him. The centurion had recognized that Christ was living in direct submission to the Father's will in the same way that he was living in submission to his superior officer. Therefore, Christ had authority to *command the healing* in the *same way* the centurion could command soldiers. Christ praised this spiritual insight of the Roman centurion. Here is the second half of this story:

> *Now when Jesus heard this, He marveled, and said to those who were following, "Truly I say to you, I have not found such great faith with anyone in Israel. And I say to you, that many shall come from east and west, and recline at the table with Abraham, and Isaac, and Jacob, in the kingdom of*

heaven; but the sons of the kingdom shall be cast out into the outer darkness; in that place there shall be weeping and gnashing of teeth." And Jesus said to the centurion, "Go your way; let it be done to you as you have believed." And the servant was healed that very hour. Matthew 8:10-13

In light of the fact that Christ said the centurion had great faith, this passage has some important things to consider about the supernatural ministry's relationship with faith.

- *Now when Jesus heard this, He marveled, and said to those who were following, "Truly I say to you, I have not found such great faith with anyone in Israel..."*

Christ *marveled* at the centurion's *faith*. The centurion had suggested an alternative way of healing his servant. The centurion *believed* that all Christ had to do was to *speak the word* for the servant to be healed. In other words, Christ need not be present. The healing could be done at a distance.

Christ *endorsed* this particular way of the centurion's thinking and believing by two things. First, the fact that the servant was actually healed at a distance endorses the centurion's viewpoint. Secondly, Christ strongly approved of the centurion by saying he had *great faith*. Christ's next words also strongly *endorse* the centurion's theology.

Two Incidents of Great Faith

- *And Jesus said to the centurion, "Go your way; let it be done to you as you have believed." And the servant was healed that very hour.*

The centurion was in *control* of this healing. Remember that Christ's original intention was to come to the centurion's home to heal his servant. However, the centurion *changed the circumstance by his faith.* He received an *unusual miracle* for his servant at a *distance* by virtue of his faith. Christ expressed this truth by saying, *"let it be done to you as you have believed."* It was done for the centurion *as he believed.* He believed for a greater miracle and received it. Christ did not initiate the idea that He could heal at a distance. Christ was able to do that for which the centurion's faith allowed. In this case, the *great faith* of the centurion allowed for a *great miracle.*

The truth of the *believer's control* in matters of healing and miracles is often untaught and sometimes maligned by those who want to keep these matters murky for various reasons. Sometimes ministers are fearful, wanting to avoid responsibility for healing. Or they want a way to let someone who is ill or injured avoid responsibility for their own healing. In doing this, ministers seriously fail the suffering person by not teaching them the truth of this matter. This is often very shortsighted. These ministers may short-circuit the process of obtaining faith for healing. Instead of encouraging those suffering to *cry out* to the Father for *faith in Christ as Healer*, they *misplace* the responsibility back upon the Father. Therefore, the sick and injured passively remain in their conditions.

Instead of facing and confessing their own fears and failures in this matter, thereby growing in faith, these ministers may embrace an unscriptural and unbelieving doctrine that puts responsibility on a supposedly mysterious God who is revealing His will in debilitating sickness and pain. By doing this, they are not seeking to learn from, and to duplicate the ministry of the Savior who healed and delivered the hurting people whom He encountered.

The Woman Healed By Christ After Twelve Years

The three passages, Matthew 9:22-24, Mark 5:24-34 and Luke 8:42-48, concern Christ's healing of a woman with a hemorrhage of twelve years in duration. Since they are essentially the same story, we will review the most detailed of the three accounts, found in Mark's Gospel.

> *...a great multitude was following Him and pressing in on Him. And a woman who had had a hemorrhage for twelve years, and had endured much at the hands of many physicians, and had spent all that she had and was not helped at all, but rather had grown worse, after hearing about Jesus, came up in the crowd behind Him, and touched His cloak. For she thought, "If I just touch His garments, I shall get well." And immediately the flow of her blood was dried up; and she felt in her body that she was healed of her affliction. And immediately Jesus, perceiving in Himself that the power proceeding from Him had gone forth, turned around in the crowd and said, "Who touched My*

garments?" And His disciples said to Him, "You see the multitude pressing in on You, and You say, 'Who touched Me'?" And He looked around to see the woman who had done this. But the woman fearing and trembling, aware of what had happened to her, came and fell down before Him, and told Him the whole truth. And He said to her, "Daughter, your faith has made you well; go in peace, and be healed of your affliction."
Mark 5:24b-34

The following points seem important to understanding this passage.

- *...a great multitude was following Him and pressing in on Him. And a woman who had had a hemorrhage for twelve years, and had endured much at the hands of many physicians, and had spent all that she had and was not helped at all, but rather had grown worse, after hearing about Jesus, came up in the crowd behind Him, and touched His cloak...*

The detailed description of the woman seems important in this passage. She had been ill for twelve years and had become destitute in the process of trying to get well. Additionally, the passage reveals that her attempts to get well using natural means had resulted not only in destitution, but also her treatments by *physicians* caused her to *endure much* only to *grow worse*. If sickness and pain was a blessing from God, then this woman was indeed blessed. The Father obviously did not believe this woman's suffering was a blessing, nor did she. She reached out for help by pressing through the crowd around Christ from behind Him.

- *For she thought, "If I just touch His garments, I shall get well."*

Noteworthy is the fact that Mark's Gospel says *For she thought* rather than some indication that she was inspired by the Holy Spirit. She precipitated this situation of healing by *determining in her heart* that touching the garments of Christ would bring healing to her. There had been no teaching or encouragement by Christ concerning healing through His garments. This was an original thought on her part. There is no evidence of Divine inspiration of her thought. There was nothing special about Christ's clothing. This reveals the gracious nature of the God of healing. God will heal when true faith is expressed, no matter what the expression, imperfect as it may be. (The Father is not a legalist or an unrealistic perfectionist.) The Father allows believers to initiate the response to the Gospel or to the presence of Christ Himself, and will faithfully reveal Himself in healing the sick and injured.

- *And immediately the flow of her blood was dried up; and she felt in her body that she was healed of her affliction.*

This woman received what she needed from the Father. Her healing was *immediate* in this case. She also *felt in her body* that she was healed. Divine healing often will come with something to *feel*. There are common manifestations that are sometimes *felt* when someone is healed. Often the feeling of *heat,* or less occasionally the feeling of *cold,* accompanies healing. Sometimes a strong *feeling of electricity* or a less strong *tingling* accompanies the gift of miracles. Sometimes both manifestations will be present. However, none of these manifestations are actually needed to heal the sick. Some are healed and no one feels anything in particular. God commonly grants manifestations in order to communicate that healing has occurred. For the one being healed, faith in Christ as Healer comes first, then possibly manifestations, but never manifestations first, then faith.

- *And immediately Jesus, perceiving in Himself that the power proceeding from Him had gone forth...*

Not only did the woman *feel* her healing but also Jesus Himself *felt* something had happen. Jesus *perceived* that *power* had *gone forth* to heal someone. In this case, the Greek word translated *power* here comes from the common word *dunamis,* as does the word that is translated *miracle.* The word *miracle* means literally a *work of power.* Personal experience allows speculation that Christ *felt the living electricity, the Divine power of the Holy Spirit flow* from Him. Since He knew this feeling from previous miracles, He knew that someone had been healed, but was not clear who the person was.

- *...turned around in the crowd and said, "Who touched My garments?"*

This woman had come up behind Christ, so that He was not aware of her. After Christ perceived that someone had been healed, He *turned around* and spoke to the crowd to determine who the person was. It appears that Christ was *not* in control of this healing, and that He did not know who was healed. The Holy Spirit had healed this woman through Him without His prior knowledge. He had come to know that someone had been healed *during* the healing.

Christ's own faith was not directly involved in the woman's healing. The woman had *precipitated* this sequence of events and had received what she expected from God. She was, for all practical purposes, *in control* of her own healing. This becomes even more obvious as the rest of the passage is considered.

- *And His disciples said to Him, "You see the multitude pressing in on You, and You say, 'Who touched Me'?" And He looked around to see the woman who had done this.*

Christ's disciples fail to understand *what kind* of *touch* Christ is asking about. They only see that a multitude has been physically touching Him. Christ is concerned only with *one particular touch*, a *touch* that has released the Holy Spirit's power and brought healing to someone. Christ is trying to identify the person who touched Him with faith.

- *But the woman fearing and trembling, aware of what had happened to her, came and fell down before Him, and told Him the whole truth.*

Two Incidents of Great Faith

The woman reveals herself to Christ and the others. She was *aware of what had happened to her* and explains *the whole truth* to Christ, His disciples, and apparently to the whole multitude. This strongly indicates that when someone is completely healed, they will know it either by a manifestation of healing or simply by the fact of not having pain or symptoms any longer. In this situation, *both* Christ and the woman *knew immediately* that she had been healed.

- *And He said to her, "Daughter, your faith has made you well; go in peace, and be healed of your affliction."*

Christ reveals what caused this woman to be healed. It was her faith. Since Christ repeatedly tells people who have received healing that, *"your faith has made you well"*, believers ought to take this seriously. Some have reacted to this truth about faith simply because they are fearful that this condemns people who are ill. They are concerned that they may not have this kind of faith, or they argue that they had this kind of faith and were not healed. Unfortunately, this is a serious misunderstanding of the nature of faith itself. This will require detailed explanation in a future chapter. However, at present it is enough to say that these words of Christ condemn no one. In fact, Christ words are the *truth* and the *truth will set us free*. No one can afford to react negatively to the truth simply because someone has abused it in the past. Believers must rejoice in this woman's healing and agree with Christ: *Her faith has made her well.*

There seem to be four persons in this equation of healing. The four persons are the Father, Christ, the Holy Spirit, and the woman. While Christ was the focus of the woman's faith, Christ's own will was uninvolved. Christ was *unaware* of the woman until she was healed. Nor does Christ credit her healing to a sovereign God who unpredictably heals people. In fact, the Father had *already revealed* His will: The Father wants people well. The Holy Spirit administered the Father's settled will in response to the woman's faith in Christ as Healer. Christ credited the woman's *faith* in the healing. This was obviously correct as she *precipitated* the whole set of events.

There was a multitude around Christ touching Him, but this woman was the only one who was healed in this situation. She simply had faith that if she touched Christ's clothing she would be healed. The Holy Spirit responded to her faith in Christ and healed her. The Father's will was settled, Christ was essentially uninvolved, and the Holy Spirit was waiting to respond to faith in Christ. The woman was in control of her own healing. She believed and she received healing as anyone can.

Faith is Infectious and God is Gracious
The woman here thought that if she could just touch the cloak of Jesus that she would be healed. There was no indication that somehow this was a divinely inspired methodology of healing. In fact, it is apparent that she was healed, not because of her methodology but because of her faith. However, having a methodology can be helpful. In fact, the story about this woman must have been told repeatedly since many other sick people successfully

adopted this methodology of healing. In other words, the faith of the woman and the story of her healing inspired the faith of many others.

> _And wherever He entered villages, or cities, or countryside, they were laying the sick in the market places, and entreating Him that they might just touch the fringe of His cloak; and as many as touched it were being cured. Mark 6:56[1]_

The Holy Spirit continued to release healing to those who sought to touch Christ's clothing, thinking and believing that if they did so they would be healed. God is gracious and does not dictate that faith must be expressed only in one fashion in the matter of healing.

This story ought to inspire believers as well. It reveals that God is extremely gracious in this matter of healing. He is not a perfectionist waiting for believers to get everything just right. He simply wants people to believe in His goodness, His grace and His mercy expressed in the sacrifice of His Son for all. If Christians believe this, then faith for healing is relatively easy.

---

[1] _Cross Reference: Matthew 14:36_

~12~

Christ's Followers Heal Specific People

Duplicating the Ministry of Christ

Earlier in this book, the general descriptions of mass healing ministry were reviewed. In those descriptions, the twelve apostles, as well as Stephen, Philip, Paul and Barnabus, all *duplicated* the ministry of the Savior. We then reviewed the specific healing events in Christ's ministry to further discover the Father's will. This chapter is an analysis of the specific healing events by Christ's First Century followers.

Performing Miracles and Healing

Peter Heals the Lame Man at the Temple

The first specific miracle where an individual is identified as being healed by a follower of Christ is found in the Book of Acts, Chapter 3. Apparently, this event occurred only days after Pentecost. Here is the story:

> _Now Peter and John were going up to the temple at the ninth hour, the hour of prayer. And a certain man who had been lame from his mother's womb was being carried along, whom they used to set down every day at the gate of the temple which is called Beautiful, in order to beg alms of those who were entering the temple. And when he saw Peter and John about to go into the temple, he began asking to receive alms. And Peter, along with John, fixed his gaze upon him and said, "Look at us!" And he began to give them his attention, expecting to receive something from them. But Peter said, "I do not possess silver and gold, but what I do have I give to you: In the name of Jesus Christ the Nazarene-- walk!" And seizing him by the right hand, he raised him up; and immediately his feet and his ankles were strengthened. And with a leap, he stood upright and began to walk; and he entered the temple with them, walking and leaping and praising God. And all the people saw him walking and praising God... Acts 3:1-9_

This story has some similar elements that have been seen in the ministry of the Savior. Peter and John on an ordinary day were going the Temple to pray and an ordinary set of events unexpectedly turned into an extraordinary experience of God's grace.

- *Now Peter and John were going up to the temple at the ninth hour, the hour of prayer. And a certain man who had been lame from his mother's womb was being carried along, whom they used to set down every day at the gate of the temple which is called Beautiful, in order to beg alms of those who were entering the temple.*

The description of the beggar involved is somewhat detailed. This man had a birth defect that caused him to be lame. Apparently, his family brought him to the Temple's gate everyday so that he could beg for a living. This is where he encountered Peter and John.

- *And when he saw Peter and John about to go into the temple, he began asking to receive alms. And Peter, along with John, fixed his gaze upon him and said, "Look at us!" And he began to give them his attention, expecting to receive something from them.*

There does not seem to be anything extraordinary happening to this man before Peter begins to speak to him. However, as he begs alms from Peter and John, Peter takes particular notice of him. The passage says that Peter *fixed his gaze upon him*. This may indicate that Peter received revelation about this particular man. Because Peter gave this man such attention, the man thought that Peter was going to give him money.

- *But Peter said, "I do not possess silver and gold, but what I do have I give to you: In the name of Jesus Christ the Nazarene-- walk!"*

Peter was aware that the lame man thought he was going to give him money. Peter told the lame man that he did not have silver or gold to give him. What Peter said he had to give is enlightening. Peter said to him, *"what I do have I give to you..."*. Obviously, Peter believed that he had healing and miracles to give to the man. This is similar to Christ's statement after commissioning the Twelve. Christ commanded them to *cast out demons and to heal the sick*. Shortly after that Christ told them, *"freely you have received freely give."* Just as Peter said here, Christ had not given them money to give, He had given them the authority to cast out demons and to heal the sick. Peter had *freely received* the authority to heal the sick from Christ and now he was *freely giving* healing away. Believers today also have authority to heal in Christ's name and can freely give healing away. When they know this by faith, they will be able to do it. Peter acted upon his own statement and took the man by the hand.

Peter also knew that healing was *not* being done any other way than through Jesus Christ. He said to the lame man, *"In the name of Jesus Christ the Nazarene--walk!"* The healing was not done because Peter had any resident power, but because Christ had commissioned Peter to heal. Peter was then able to exercise the same kind of authority Christ did simply because he was doing it in Christ's name.

Christ's Followers Heal Specific People

Peter understood that the Father's will was to heal and deliver. Peter had come to understand this as he observed the Savior demonstrating the Father's heart in all matters for three years. He had received instruction and authority to accomplish the same things in Christ's name. Likewise, the Great Commission was given to Peter and the other apostles to instruct and commission those Christians to do these same merciful works through the authority of Jesus Christ's name. In other words, while many believers do not know it, they are _already commissioned_ to do mighty works in the name of Jesus Christ. What they need to know is _how_ to do these works. Here is what Peter did for the man.

- _And seizing him by the right hand, he raised him up; and immediately his feet and his ankles were strengthened. And with a leap, he stood upright and began to walk; and he entered the temple with them, walking and leaping and praising God. And all the people saw him walking and praising God..._

This may be another situation of _hopeful neutrality_ in faith on the part of the recipient. The lame man certainly was healed unexpectedly. It appears that Peter had an overcoming faith and may have received Divine guidance before healing this man. Peter certainly _knew_ that he _had healing to give_.

This man also represents another person who had been disabled for a long period before being healed. The length of time someone is ill or disabled certainly does not reveal the will of the Father for them. Even if they were born in that condition, the will of the Father is healing and deliverance. Even if they do not seem to have faith, the will of the Father is healing. Perhaps the Father will send someone like Peter who will *believe* for them.

Occasionally, a healing or miracle will occur in the Gospels without specific mention of believing or faith being present in the description offered. This may give a false impression that the healing or miracle was done in some other way. In the case of Peter healing the lame man at the Temple's gate, this is true. The description of the healing has nothing at all to say about faith. If one simply studied the account without reference to the teaching that Christ did about faith throughout His healing ministry, then someone could suggest that faith had nothing to do with this healing. However, this would be incorrect. In fact, Peter himself describes what happened to this man to the witnesses of this man's healing. This is what Peter says is responsible for this healing:

> *And on the basis of faith in His name, it is the name of Jesus which has strengthened this man whom you see and know; and the faith which comes through Him has given him this perfect health in the presence of you all. Acts 3:16*

Since the healed man was expecting money and not healing, Peter is saying that *his (Peter's) faith* in the name of Jesus is what enabled him to heal this man. How does someone work the works of God? Miracles and healing are performed by faith in Jesus Christ as Healer and Deliverer.

Peter Heals Aeneas at Lydda

A second specific healing involving Peter occurs in the Book of Acts, Chapter 9. This happened shortly after the conversion of Saul, who became the apostle Paul. This is the story:

> _Now it came about that as Peter was traveling through all those parts, he came down also to the saints who lived at Lydda. And there he found a certain man named Aeneas, who had been bedridden eight years, for he was paralyzed. And Peter said to him, "Aeneas, Jesus Christ heals you; arise, and make your bed." And immediately he arose. And all who lived at Lydda and Sharon saw him, and they turned to the Lord. Acts 9:32-35_

Again, the Savior's ministry is revealed in Peter. Peter arrived in Lydda to minister to the believers there. Peter there encountered a bedridden man named Aeneas who may have been a believer.

- _Now it came about that as Peter was traveling through all those parts, he came down also to the saints who lived at Lydda. And there he found a certain man named Aeneas, who had been bedridden eight years, for he was paralyzed._

Aeneas had been paralyzed and bedridden for eight years. This was no indication that the Father wanted him to remain that way. Peter thought otherwise and acted out what he believed.

- *And Peter said to him, "Aeneas, Jesus Christ heals you; arise, and make your bed." And immediately he arose. And all who lived at Lydda and Sharon saw him, and they turned to the Lord.*

Peter was clear about who was doing the actual healing. He told Aeneas, *"Jesus Christ heals you."* Peter was clear that any healing coming through him was simply the Savior making Himself known through His Bride, the Church. Peter knew that it was *Christ in him the hope of glory[1]* that was manifesting the Father's works. There is no indication of Divine guidance in this matter. Peter was just acting out of his faith in Jesus Christ and the Father was doing His works. This seems much like the Savior.

Peter Raises Tabitha from the Dead
The story of Peter's ministry in that region continues without a break in the Acts of the Apostles. However, this city is now Joppa, a city near Lydda where the former healing took place. In fact, as this story begins, Peter is still in Lydda.

> *Now in Joppa there was a certain disciple named Tabitha (which translated in Greek is called Dorcas); this woman was abounding with deeds of kindness and charity, which she continually did. And it came about at that time that she fell sick and died; and when they had washed her body, they laid it in an upper room. And since Lydda was near Joppa, the disciples, having heard that Peter was there, sent two men to him, entreating him, "Do not*

---

[1] Colossians 1:27

delay to come to us." And Peter arose and went with them. And when he had come, they brought him into the upper room; and all the widows stood beside him weeping, and showing all the tunics and garments that Dorcas used to make while she was with them. But Peter sent them all out and knelt down and prayed, and turning to the body, he said, "Tabitha, arise." And she opened her eyes, and when she saw Peter, she sat up. And he gave her his hand and raised her up; and calling the saints and widows, he presented her alive. And it became known all over Joppa, and many believed in the Lord. Acts 9:36-42

This resurrection has several elements that are reminiscent of Christ's ministry.

- *Now in Joppa there was a certain disciple named Tabitha (which translated in Greek is called Dorcas); this woman was abounding with deeds of kindness and charity, which she continually did. And it came about at that time that she fell sick and died; and when they had washed her body, they laid it in an upper room.*

Luke described this particular Christian woman's character in a very positive sense. Apparently, she was well known for her deeds. While Peter was in the region, she became sick and died. Her body had been washed and placed in an upper room. This would have been the first step in preparation of Tabitha for burial.

Performing Miracles and Healing

- *And since Lydda was near Joppa, the disciples, having heard that Peter was there, sent two men to him, entreating him, "Do not delay to come to us."*

The Christians that lived in Joppa knew that Peter was there. Perhaps they had heard of Aeneas' recent healing. Perhaps, they remembered that Peter's shadow had healed many. They knew the Savior's ministry was being *duplicated* in Peter. They saw the opportunity for a resurrection and sent two believers to him to ask him to come and pray for Tabitha. They understood that time was critical and that Tabitha would need to be buried soon. Peter responded to their request and their obvious faith.

- *And Peter arose and went with them. And when he had come, they brought him into the upper room; and all the widows stood beside him weeping, and showing all the tunics and garments that Dorcas used to make while she was with them. But Peter sent them all out and knelt down and prayed...*

Peter was brought into the room where Tabitha's body had been placed. The room was full of people mourning over Tabitha's death and remembering her ability as a seamstress. This ability may be how Tabitha showed the *good deeds* and *charity* that the earlier verses mentioned.

In actions much like the Savior, Peter makes everyone leave the room. This is much like the Savior. On several occasions, Christ made people leave the room before praying for someone, or He took them to another location to pray for them, away from the crowd. After the room was empty, Peter knelt down and prayed.

- *...and turning to the body, he said, "Tabitha, arise." And she opened her eyes, and when she saw Peter, she sat up. And he gave her his hand and raised her up; and calling the saints and widows, he presented her alive. And it became known all over Joppa, and many believed in the Lord.*

The Savior, on several previous occasions, had described *death* as *sleeping.* Those situations resulted in resurrections by Christ simply speaking to the dead person as if He were waking them from sleep. In this case, Peter seemed to be doing the same thing. Peter simply told Tabitha to *get up.* After Tabitha got up, Peter presented her to those who had been mourning her.

Paul Heals the Lame Man at Lystra

Earlier in this book, we reviewed of the numerous general statements of the healing ministry of Paul. The lame man in this next story is the first individual that Scripture describes as being healed by the apostle Paul. Here is the story:

...and there they (Paul and Barnabus) continued to preach the gospel. And at Lystra there was sitting a certain man, without strength in his feet, lame from his mother's womb, who had never walked. This man was listening to Paul as he spoke, who, when he had fixed his gaze upon him, and had seen that he had faith to be made well, said with a loud voice,

Performing Miracles and Healing

_"Stand upright on your feet". And he leaped up and
began to walk. And when the multitudes saw what
Paul had done, they raised their voice, saying in the
Lycaonian language, ""The gods have become like
men and have come down to us." and saying, "Men,
why are you doing these things? We are also men of
the same nature as you, and preach the gospel to
you in order that you should turn from these vain
things to a living God..." Acts 14:7-15a_

This healing miracle occurred as Paul and Barnabus
traveled in ministry and preached the Gospel.

* _...and there they (Paul and Barnabus) continued to
preach the gospel. And at Lystra there was sitting a
certain man, without strength in his feet, lame from his
mother's womb, who had never walked. This man was
listening to Paul as he spoke..._

Much like the Savior's ministry, deliverance,
healing and miracles followed when Paul and Barnabus
preached the Gospel of Christ. Their objective was
obviously to proclaim Christ in such a way to produce faith
in Christ as Savior, Healer, Deliverer and Lord. In this
context, Paul and Barnabus encountered a lame man as
they preached the Gospel. This lame man was listening to
Paul as he preached Christ and Paul began to notice him
and perceive that the man had faith to be made well.

* _This man was listening to Paul as he spoke, who, when
he had fixed his gaze upon him, and had seen that he
had faith to be made well said with a loud voice, "Stand_

274

upright on your feet." And he leaped up and began to walk.

What indicated to Paul that this man had faith which would enable him to be made well is not entirely evident. The passage says Paul *had seen* that the man had faith to be made well. Perhaps, Paul received a discerning revelation which made him *see* that the man could be healed. In any case, Paul boldly commanded the man to get up. When the man got up, he was entirely well. This caused quite a stir among the people in this locality.

- *And when the multitudes saw what Paul had done, they raised their voice, saying in the Lycaonian language, "The gods have become like men and have come down to us." and saying, "Men, why are you doing these things? We are also men of the same nature as you, and preach the gospel to you in order that you should turn from these vain things to a living God...*

These people thought Paul and Barnabus were gods. Paul did not let this wrong perception of them go unchallenged. He immediately told them that he and Barnabus were ordinary men with the *same nature* as they had. Paul put the healing into the context that these people should turn from idols to a living God who had come in the form of Christ and had now healed this man. Today, a few would like to be seen as *gods* because they heal the sick. However, anyone healing or doing miracles is a man or woman with the *same nature* as everyone else. This is why *every believer* is a candidate to be used by the Father to heal the suffering.

Paul Raises Eutychus from the Dead

A resurrection from the dead is also found in Paul's ministry. In the ordinary context of his preaching and teaching ministry, Paul raised a boy from the dead. This is the story:

> *And on the first day of the week, when we were gathered together to break bread, Paul began talking to them, intending to depart the next day, and he prolonged his message until midnight. And there were many lamps in the upper room where we were gathered together. And there was a certain young man named Eutychus sitting on the window sill, sinking into a deep sleep; and as Paul kept on talking, he was overcome by sleep and fell down from the third floor, and was picked up dead. But Paul went down and fell upon him and after embracing him, he said, "Do not be troubled, for his life is in him." And when he had gone back up, and had broken the bread and eaten, he talked with them a long while, until daybreak, and so departed. And they took away the boy alive, and were greatly comforted. Acts 20:7-12*

This story begins with Paul extending his message to these believers because he was leaving the next day. The hour became late and the setting reflected that.

- *And on the first day of the week, when we were gathered together to break bread, Paul began talking to them, intending to depart the next day, and he prolonged his message until midnight. And there were many lamps in the upper room where we were gathered together.*

Any Church that has had extended meetings that have gone late into the night understands what happened here. A boy sitting in a window, where it probably was cooler, fell soundly asleep during Paul's lengthy message and fell out of the window. This would be rather humorous except for the fact that the meeting was being held in an third story upper room and the boy was killed by the fall.

- *And there was a certain young man named Eutychus sitting on the window sill, sinking into a deep sleep; and as Paul kept on talking, he was overcome by sleep and fell down from the third floor, and was picked up dead.*

Paul immediately responded to this crisis by coming down to where the boy was laying and embracing him. Paul then declared to the observers that the boy was alive. It is very possible that the boy's parents were in that group.

- *But Paul went down and fell upon him and after embracing him, he said, "Do not be troubled, for his life is in him." And when he had gone back up, and had broken the bread and eaten, he talked with them a long while, until daybreak, and so departed. And they took away the boy alive, and were greatly comforted*

The boy not only was not dead but was uninjured. It seems from the various resurrections that have been found in Christ's and His followers' ministries that healing is always a part of a resurrection. In other words, whatever caused the death is no longer a problem when the resurrection occurs. This is the reason that resurrections must be considered in any teaching on healing.

It appears that resurrections may be less common than healings, but not any more difficult from the perspective of the one raising the dead. Believers must recognize this possibility without acting in extreme ways and trying to force their own will on other people who are not prepared to believe. The matter of a deceased loved one should be in the hands of the family members. Their perceptions of what should be done should be foremost. Guidance from local Church governmental leadership should be considered. Everyone else should quietly and kindly submit to the conclusions of the family. If an unusual faith arises in the family members and an invitation is given to a particular anointed servant of God for prayer, then potentially a resurrection can come out of these events. As a rule of thumb, all resurrections in the New Testament came within moments of the time that the servant of God arrived and prayed.[2] No one should ever torment a family by days of waiting.

Paul's Snake-bite Miracle
While essentially not a situation involving the ministry of healing, Paul's personal experience with being bitten by a poisonous snake is revealing. Here is the story that is found in the last chapter of Acts of the Apostles.

---

[2] Of course, the resurrection of Christ is a different kind of resurrection.

...the island was called Malta. And the natives showed us extraordinary kindness; for because of the rain that had set in and because of the cold, they kindled a fire and received us all. But when Paul had gathered a bundle of sticks and laid them on the fire, a viper came out because of the heat, and fastened on his hand. And when the natives saw the creature hanging from his hand, they began saying to one another, "Undoubtedly this man is a murderer, and though he has been saved from the sea, justice has not allowed him to live." However he shook the creature off into the fire and suffered no harm. But they were expecting that he was about to swell up or suddenly fall down dead. But after they had waited a long time and had seen nothing unusual happen to him, they changed their minds and began to say that he was a god. Acts 28:1b-6

After God had given Paul grace to live, without any harm, after a shipwreck, a viper bit Paul in front of a group of island people.

- *...But when Paul had gathered a bundle of sticks and laid them on the fire, a viper came out because of the heat, and fastened on his hand. And when the natives saw the creature hanging from his hand, they began saying to one another, "Undoubtedly this man is a murderer, and though he has been saved from the sea, justice has not allowed him to live."*

Performing Miracles and Healing

The natives of this island assumed that Paul must be under some sort of judgement because of this set of events. However Paul reacted much differently than they expected.

- _However he shook the creature off into the fire and suffered no harm. But they were expecting that he was about to swell up or suddenly fall down dead. But after they had waited a long time and had seen nothing unusual happen to him, they changed their minds and began to say that he was a god._

The Divine protection of Paul from this kind of harm became evident to these people. There is no evidence of any kind of desperate prayer by Paul. The account suggests that Paul did not act as if there was a problem. He reacted much like the Savior would in such a circumstance. He knew that the will of the Father was for him to _finish his course_. Therefore, he could believe for a protective healing for himself.

Paul Heals the Father of Publius

The final healing event in the Acts of the Apostles occurs right after the events surrounding Paul's snakebite. In fact, the text hints that this event opened the door for Paul to minister to a leading family on the island. This is the story:

> _Now in the neighborhood of that place were lands belonging to the leading man of the island, named Publius, who welcomed us and entertained us courteously three days. And it came about that the father of Publius was lying in bed afflicted with_

recurrent fever and dysentery; and Paul went in to see him and after he had prayed, he laid his hands on him and healed him. And after this had happened, the rest of the people on the island who had diseases were coming to him and getting cured. Acts 28:7-9

The man had some sort or recurrent fever and dysentery. This healing in turn caused people to believe that Paul could help them and they came to him.

Paul successfully laid hands on and prayed for the father of Publius, who was the leading man of the island. The account says that Paul *healed him.* Many in the Church today probably would react to this if it were not in the Bible. Someone would want to immediately correct anyone saying they had healed the sick. While the Bible says repeatedly that the disciples healed the sick, the culture of the western church is uncomfortable with this. Out of some misguided desire for humility, they want the individual doing the healing to be left out of the equation, although the Bible gives them credit. Of course, everyone knows that it is because of Christ that this healing was possible. However, it was Paul, the apostle of Christ used to do the healing.

In order to perform healing and miracles consistently, the issue of humility must be dealt with. For most people, *false humility* is a larger barrier to performing healing and miracles than pride. Many believers are afraid of presumption. They are afraid of pride. They are afraid that trying to perform healing and miracles might not show humility. Because the culture of the modern Church has often fed these unscriptural attitudes, many are afraid to try and many will not boldly proclaim what Christ will do through them.

In many churches today, *caution* is much more valued in believers than *boldness* for Christ. Caution in matters of healing and miracles is often seen as wise and boldness is seen as shallow and presumptive. Of course, Christ has *nothing* to say about presumption, and has given a great deal of encouragement for bold faith. Every believer ought to be praying to the Father to grow in bold faith in witnessing and supernatural works for Jesus Christ. Every leader ought to be encouraging the people of God to boldness, especially when they make mistakes. The Father will often honor *the mistake* that is done *boldly* in Christ's name. There is no other way for the people of God to learn to perform miracles and healing. Everyone must start somewhere. The people of God must be allowed to make honest mistakes and thereby grow in their knowledge of a faithful Father. The needs of the last days harvest demand that the people of God have opportunity to learn to use the *supernatural equipment* of the gifts of healings and miracles.

Section 3

Formulating a Christ-Centered Theology of Healing

~13~

Preaching the Gospel with Signs Following

Called to Perform Two Activities

The Lord Jesus demonstrated in His own ministry that if a servant of Christ wants to have a Christ-like ministry, he ought to do two different but related activities. The servant wishing to emulate the Savior must *teach* and *preach*.

> *...He (Christ) departed from there to teach and preach in their cities. Matthew 11:1b*

The apostle Paul encouraged Timothy to duplicate the Savior's ministry by doing both activities.

> *...teach and preach these principles.*
> *1 Timothy 6:2b*

The apostle Paul also encouraged Timothy about these two kinds of activities that would cause some governmental leaders to be worthy of honor.

> *Let the elders who rule well be counted worthy of double honor, especially those who work hard at preaching and teaching. 1 Timothy 5:17*

Preaching the Gospel with the attesting signs of healing and miracles must take priority and is foundational to good teaching. However, teaching is also very important. No teaching ministry should ever be considered as unimportant or simply as offering information. Anointed teaching imparts revelation about the whole counsel of God. Teaching imparts biblical truth in a systematic way. Proper teaching is the backbone to discipleship and is the preventative to deception. A properly taught person is very difficult to deceive. The apostle Paul, who teaches a great deal about the importance of preaching, reveals in several places that he was also appointed as a *teacher*.

> *...I was appointed a preacher and an apostle...and as a teacher of the Gentiles in faith and truth. 1 Timothy 2:7*

The apostle Paul reminded Timothy again in his second letter of his dual call as a preacher and teacher.

> *...I was appointed a preacher and an apostle and a teacher. 2 Timothy 1:11*

What is the distinction between preaching and teaching? Most people could probably draw good distinctions between preaching and teaching out of their own experiences. They might suggest that preaching and teaching concern the style of presentation. This may be true. However, it is better to allow the New Testament to show how it draws distinctions between these two important activities.

The Gospel of Christ and His Kingdom

It appears that the first distinction is the message. Preaching is often connected to the Gospel, the good news about the Lord Jesus Christ and the Kingdom of God. Teaching is not always identified as closely with this message. For example, where teaching and proclamation (preaching) are mentioned together in Scripture, the subject of teaching may be often unspecified. However, this is not so of proclamation.

> _And Jesus ...teaching in their synagogues, and proclaiming the Gospel of the kingdom, and healing... Matthew 4:23a (CR: Matthew 9:35)_

Again, this is often found where the two activities are mentioned together. The subject of teaching is often unspecified but the subject of preaching is often mentioned.

> _...He (Jesus) was teaching the people in the temple and preaching the Gospel... Luke 20:1a_

Performing Miracles and Healing

Luke tells us something very similar. The apostles early in the Book of Acts proclaim the Gospel about Jesus Christ. The subject of teaching is unspecified, but this is not true of their proclamation.

> ...*being greatly disturbed because they were teaching the people and proclaiming in Jesus the resurrection from the dead. Acts 4:2*

Surveying the book of Acts shows that the message which had attesting supernatural signs was the message of the Gospel. However, this simple Gospel message was ordinarily *preached* rather than taught. While the message of teaching was often unspecified, this is not always true. For instance, Luke reports what the Twelve were preaching and teaching.

> ...*they (the twelve apostles) kept right on teaching and preaching Jesus as the Christ. Acts 5:42*

Proclamation or preaching is concerning Jesus Christ. In this case, teaching revealed Jesus as the Christ. Paul tells us the same thing in Colossians. Preachers are to proclaim *Him*. However, we may *teach wisdom* to every man. This implies slightly greater latitude in teaching that does not exist in true biblical preaching.

> *And we proclaim Him, admonishing every man and teaching every man with all wisdom, that we may present every man complete in Christ.*
> *Colossians 1:28*

Luke reports that Paul and Barnabus also did the two activities. However, there is no strong distinction apparent in this passage.

> _...Paul and Barnabas...teaching and preaching, ...the word of the Lord. Acts 15:35_

The message that Paul and Barnabus were preaching and teaching was the _word of the Lord._ The word _Lord_ in this verse is a reference to the _Lord Jesus Christ._ They were proclaiming and teaching about the Lord Jesus Christ. In another reference about the ministry of the apostle Paul, his ministry is revealed in these two activities while imprisoned in his rented quarters in Rome.

> _(Paul)...preaching the kingdom of God, and teaching concerning the Lord Jesus Christ..._
> _Acts 28:31b_

In this case, Luke reveals that Paul was preaching the Gospel of the Kingdom of God and teaching about Christ.

In summary, preaching always seems connected with the simple Gospel of Jesus Christ and the Kingdom of God. In some contrast, teaching is about Christ as well but may allow additional latitude and perhaps more depth. The miraculous attestation of God seems only connected in Scripture to preaching the Gospel, however.

> _And He (Christ) sent them (the Twelve) out to proclaim the kingdom of God, and to perform healing... And departing, they (the Twelve) began_

going about among the villages, preaching the gospel, and healing everywhere. Luke 9:2, 6

Preaching the Gospel of Christ

The focus of the ministry of the apostle Paul was to preach the Gospel of Christ.

For Christ did not send me to baptize, but to preach the Gospel, not in cleverness of speech, that the cross of Christ should not be made void. For the word of the cross is to those who are perishing foolishness, but to us who are being saved it is the power of God. 1 Corinthians 1:17-18

Paul's words certainly have great application in our day. Consider what Paul says about the preaching the Gospel:

- _...Christ...(sent me)...to preach the Gospel, not in cleverness of speech, that the cross of Christ should not be made void._

Paul tells us that he purposely avoided _cleverness of speech_ so that a simple message about the cross might be preached. Paul was concerned that somehow the simple message about the cross might be _made void_ by the complexities of doctrinal teaching. He intimately connects _the word of the cross_ to preaching the Gospel. The cross will always be prominent in true preaching of the Gospel.

- _For the word of the cross is to those who are perishing foolishness, but to us who are being saved it is the power of God._

Paul also tells us that this type of simple preaching is to the _saved_ the _power of God._ In other words, the preaching of the cross releases the power of God in the lives of believers. The Holy Spirit produces the things that the cross purchases in the lives of those who believe the Gospel. Minimally, those things produced in the life of believers should include forgiveness, healing and deliverance from evil. A few verses later in 1 Corinthians, Paul continues his explanation of the importance of keeping the Gospel simple:

> _And when I came to you, brethren, I did not come with superiority of speech or of wisdom, proclaiming to you the testimony of God. For I determined to know nothing among you except Jesus Christ, and Him crucified. And I was with you in weakness and in fear and in much trembling. And my message and my preaching were not in persuasive words of wisdom, but in demonstration of the Spirit and of power, that your faith should not rest on the wisdom of men, but on the power of God.. 1 Corinthians 2:1-5_

Paul's words are remarkable in their clarity and application in this day. Consider these thoughts:

- _And when I came to you, brethren, I did not come with superiority of speech or of wisdom, proclaiming to you the testimony of God._

Paul continues the same line of thought on the need for simplicity in proclamation of the Gospel. Paul writes that he did not seek for the eloquence of a _superiority of speech_ in his preaching. Nor did Paul seek to present _wisdom_ coming from a greater and deeper revelation. While Paul understood these deeper things, he understood that their presentation was not the Gospel.

- _For I determined to know nothing among you except Jesus Christ, and Him crucified._

Instead, Paul focused upon a simple proclamation of Christ and the value of His cross. He reveals the results of this Christ-centered focus.

- _And my message and my preaching were not in persuasive words of wisdom, but in demonstration of the Spirit and of power..._

Again, Paul tells us that he was not looking to human wisdom to convince people of the truth about Jesus Christ. Paul implies that human wisdom tends to create complexity that inhibits faith and, therefore, limits God's power to help people. Preachers often yield to their need to be accepted by attempting to impress others with their wisdom. They often begin to preach and teach things that are not essentially the Gospel, and do not keep Christ central in their message, either in preaching or teaching. In doing so, they limit God's ability to help others. In Paul's ministry, _the Spirit demonstrated_ His _power_ to convict and convince of the realities of Christ because Paul chose to keep the Gospel simple and focused on the Savior.

- *...that your faith should not rest on the wisdom of men, but on the power of God.*

Faith again is an important issue. Faith either will *rest* on the *wisdom of men* or on the *power of God.* Paul assumes that *all* will have *faith.* Faith's *resting-place* is the issue. Faith must have an object. Faith must rest on something. Paul's phrase provides an excellent *test* of where *faith* is *resting.* If a ministry does not have an ongoing expression of the supernatural *power* of God producing scriptural signs of salvation, then that faith is likely *resting* on the *wisdom of men* in some degree. The ministry may greatly believe in the power of God, but because of acceptance of the wisdom of men on certain essential issues, it might find itself relatively powerless. If scriptural supernatural signs accompany a ministry regularly, with healing and deliverance from evil spirits, then that ministry is likely *resting* more on the *power of God* than on the wisdom of men.

In another important passage, the apostle Paul writes some additional important truths to us concerning the Gospel.

For I am not ashamed of the Gospel, for it is the power of God for salvation to everyone who believes, to the Jew first and also to the Greek. Romans 1:16

This is an important truth worth considering in more detail. An expansion of the ideas present in this verse will be helpful.

> *...it (the Gospel, the good news about Christ) is the power (the ability, the dynamic) of God working to produce salvation (eternal life, forgiveness of sins, deliverance from evil, healing, etc.) in every one who believes...* [1]

Paul explains that the dynamic which produces *salvation in all its forms* is a *believing response* to the *Gospel about Jesus Christ*. This chart simplifies the responsibilities on the human and Divine side of the relationship in ministry.

RESPONSIBILITIES	
GOD	**US**
PRODUCE SALVATION	PREACH GOSPEL
RELEASE POWER	BELIEVE GOSPEL

The chart divides the verse Romans 1:16 into component parts. It shows the responsibilities of God and the believer in the equation of salvation. On the human side of this equation, the real Gospel about Jesus Christ and His cross must be preached boldly with faith. Then those who hear must respond in faith. Preachers and believers have no responsibility to release power or to produce salvation. These things are on the Divine side of the equation. However, true faith, real believing in the Gospel on the human side of the equation, will result in God fulfilling His responsibilities. God will release the

---

[1] *Sapp's Expansive Translation of Romans 1:16*

power of the Holy Spirit which will produce the salvation things that Christ has purchased at the cross.

For the sake of clarity and simplicity, the chart above is modified to focus upon healing.

RESPONSIBILITIES	
GOD	*US*
PRODUCE HEALING	PREACH THE HEALER
RELEASE POWER	BELIEVE IN THE HEALER

As preachers proclaim, with faith and boldness, Christ as Healer, then many of those who hear will respond in faith. Preachers must resolve their own doubts and preach in faith. In turn, God will fulfill His portion of the equation drawn from Romans 1:16. The Holy Spirit's power will produce salvation in the form of healing for those that heard the Gospel and responded by believing. The preacher and the hearers have no responsibility in producing healing other than believing. Understanding this removes fear and ensures that God will receive the glory.

Distinctions between Preaching and Teaching

Unfortunately, the preaching of the complete Gospel which includes Jesus as the Crucified and Resurrected Savior, the Lord, the Healer, the Deliverer and Coming King, is often missing in modern churches. What seems to have replaced preaching the Gospel of Christ in many of these churches is a proclamation of human wisdom or a focus on teaching the Bible. The proper preaching of the Gospel of Christ brings people to faith. Teaching, on the other hand, produces understanding but does not save, heal or deliver. Unfortunately, human wisdom generally explains logically why a believer should not believe and why the supernatural power of God is not reliable.

Teaching is important and necessary, but cannot replace the bold proclamation of the Gospel with scriptural signs following. Teaching must take a secondary role. In fact, teaching cannot be what it should be without preaching first releasing the supernatural. The atmosphere for teaching will be wrong without the foundation of the preaching of the Gospel. The Gospel must be preached boldly in faith that Jesus saves, heals and delivers. The dynamic of God will produce those biblical manifestations of the Holy Spirit in those who believe what they hear.

Believers must be taught but not as a substitute for a bold proclamation of the Gospel with signs following. The bolder the preaching, the greater the signs that follow. Some have desired deliverance, healing and miracles while being unwilling to risk a public proclamation that Jesus in fact heals, delivers and does miracles. They are waiting for God to do something He has already done. In contrast, God is waiting for them to courageously preach the Gospel and perform healing. They are waiting for Divine permission when the command to do these things has already been given.

There are few unbelievers hearing a bold but simple message that Jesus will save them from sin and give them eternal life. Many leaders no longer see the wisdom in the simplicity of the Gospel. They see the Gospel as *milk* and not as *meat*. They generally overestimate the maturity of their congregations and offer too much *meat* in their Sunday morning meetings. Because they do not often present Jesus Christ as Savior, Healer and Deliverer, they seldom see new people in their meetings. God sends the unsaved where they can hear and believe the Gospel, and *see* a demonstration of the power of God to save, heal and deliver. If there is no place where an unbeliever might see a demonstration of healing and deliverance, then God sends them to a place where they might at least hear the simple Gospel and see a demonstration of God's power to save the lost. This explains why the average Baptist Church sees regular conversions to Christ, and therefore grows by evangelism, but the average charismatic congregation seldom sees growth by conversion. Instead, the average charismatic congregation teaches on Sunday morning and grows by transfer growth, if it grows at all.

Thankfully, the Church throughout the world is in a time of transition. The Holy Spirit is adjusting the Church, so that she will be like her Savior. The Father is hearing intercession from many who see the need. Therefore, the Church will come to rediscover the power of the Gospel. The Church will be triumphant as she rediscovers the supernatural power of God exhibited through preaching the Gospel of Christ as Savior, Lord, Healer and Deliverer. Powerful stirrings are being seen all over the world as the Church returns to her scriptural destiny to be like Christ and bring in the final harvest of the lost.

~14~

Healing is an Aspect of Salvation

The Meaning of "Saved"

The Greek words that are translated *salvation* and *saved* in most English versions of the Bible are a form of the common Greek word *sozo*. Forms of this word are used more than 100 times in the New Testament. This word is pregnant with meaning. It is impossible to express this Greek word's full meaning in a single English word. In fact, most English translators will use *several different words* to express *the same forms* of *sozo* in various passages.

When some churches and ministries use the word *saved* or *salvation*, they mean the initial evidences of a relationship with God such as the forgiveness of sins and regeneration. This is sometimes expressed as being *born again*. This is a biblically correct meaning but narrowly limits the biblical meaning of this Greek word. These churches under-emphasize the rest of the meaning of this word. The rest of the meaning of the word has to do with the earthly aspects of salvation. In fact, the earthly experience of salvation that includes deliverance and healing is how the Greek word for salvation is most often used in the New Testament. *Deliverance* is Christ *saving* the believer from demonic activity. *Healing* is Christ *saving* the believer from sickness and injury. Because some churches under-emphasize these earthly aspects of salvation, these churches make it difficult for those exposed to their teaching to see salvation as being anything unrelated to going to Heaven when they die.

The full meaning of this Greek word includes much more than just being *born again* and going to Heaven. The full meaning of *sozo* includes *healing* and *deliverance* from evil spirits. For instance, often when Jesus would heal persons, He would say to them *your faith has healed you.* In this case, the word *healed* would be a form of the same Greek word *sozo.* Jesus after casting out a demon would sometimes say *your faith has delivered you* or *your faith has set you free*. In these cases, a form of *sozo* would be translated *delivered* or *set free*. The basic truth about this word is this:

> The Greek word translated *saved* means much more than just going to Heaven. It means and is sometimes translated as *healed, cured, delivered, set free, made whole, preserved*, and a host of other related things. In other words, Salvation is for the here and now, as well as for eternity, and includes God's provision for all human needs.

Healing is an Aspect of Salvation

There are eighteen places in the Greek New Testament where a form of the Greek word *sozo* is used in direct reference to some sort of healing. While *sozo* is not the only Greek word that is used to describe healing, it is highly significant that forms of *sozo* are used so many times. No theology of healing can properly ignore the repeated usage of *sozo* in passages describing healing.

Before this chapter considers the implications of the usage of *sozo*, it seems appropriate to list the eighteen places where it is used and discuss them briefly. These passages are not listed in the order that they appear in the New Testament. These passages are organized around the various stories that contain them. Some stories presented here have only one usage of a form of *sozo*, some stories have many more. Here are the *eighteen* places where a form of *sozo* is used in reference to healing.

The Centurion's Slave
Jesus is encouraged to come heal a centurion's slave. In this case, a form of *sozo* is used in reference to healing. Jesus is asked to *save* the life of the slave by *healing* him.

> *And a certain centurion's slave, who was highly regarded by him, was sick and about to die. And when he heard about Jesus, he sent some Jewish elders asking Him to come and **save** (diasozo) the life of his slave. And when they had come to Jesus, they earnestly entreated Him, saying, "He is worthy for You to grant this to him..." And when those who*

had been sent returned to the house, they found the slave in good health. Luke 7:1-4, 10

Salvation is revealed as *healing* in this passage. The same form of the word *sozo* is also being used in reference to healing in another passage in the gospels. This specific Greek word, *diasozo,* means literally *to make thoroughly whole*[1] in the passage above and the one that follows. While the translators correctly chose to use the word *save* in the above passage, they could have properly translated the verse as *come and make (him) thoroughly whole* as well.

Healing Through Touching Christ's Clothing

This same form of the word *sozo* is found in this verse that describes the group of people that received healing by touching the fringe of Christ's cloak.

*...and they began to entreat Him that they might just touch the fringe of His cloak; and as many as touched it **were cured** (diasozo). Matthew 14:36*

Those who touched the fringe of Christ's cloak *were cured.* The Savior made them *thoroughly whole.* As it did then, the Savior's *salvation* today includes making people *thoroughly whole.* Mark also reveals this wonderful phenomenon with Christ's clothing.

---

[1] *diasozo "to make thoroughly whole".* There are two more references that use this particular word that do not specifically apply to healing: Acts 27:43, 1 Peter 3:20.

Healing is an Aspect of Salvation

> _And wherever He entered villages, or cities, or countryside, they were laying the sick in the market places, and entreating Him that they might just touch the fringe of His cloak; and as many as touched it **were being cured** (sozo). Mark 6:56_

These passages reveal three uses of a form of _sozo_. The next story will reveal a great number of uses.

Woman with a Twelve Year Hemorrhage

The fourth place where one form of _sozo_ is used in the New Testament is the story of the woman who was ill with a hemorrhage for twelve years. This story is one of the most frequently recorded healings in the Bible and is found in the Gospels of Matthew, Mark and Luke. The popularity of the story may also have been the reason why the events discussed above happened. People may have been inspired to touch Christ's cloak because they heard her story. In the three passages describing what Christ did for this woman, a form of _sozo_ is found six times and is consistently translated _made well_ by the translators of the New American Standard Version. For instance, Matthew uses a form of _sozo_ three times in these verses:

> _...for she was saying to herself, "If I only touch His garment, I **shall get well** (sozo)." But Jesus turning and seeing her said, "Daughter, take courage; your faith **has made you well** (sozo)." And at once the woman **was made well** (sozo). Matthew 9:21-22_

Matthew's account is very similar to Mark's account. Both accounts reveal that Christ's _salvation also includes_

303

healing. Both accounts reveal that Christ gave credit to the woman's *faith* as the reason she received *salvation* in the form of *healing*. There are two uses of *sozo* in these verses. This brings the total to eight uses in the New Testament with the two more included here:

> *For she thought, "If I just touch His garments, I* **shall get well** *(sozo)...And He (Christ) said to her, "Daughter, your faith* **has made you well** *(sozo); go in peace, and be healed of your affliction."*
> *Mark 5:28, 34*

Not surprisingly in Luke's description of the same events another form of *sozo* is found. The woman's *faith* also takes on the same importance as in the other passages.

> *And He said to her, "Daughter, your faith has* **made you well** *(sozo); go in peace."* *Luke 8:48*

This totals nine places where a form of *sozo* has been used.

The Resurrection of Jairus' Daughter

There are two places in the Gospel accounts where the Synagogue leader, Jairus, asks Jesus to heal his dying daughter. A form of *sozo* is found in both places and both are clearly references to healing. In Mark's Gospel, Jairus asks Jesus to lay His hands on his daughter that she *may get well*. Salvation is revealed as healing again.

> *...and entreated Him earnestly, saying, "My little daughter is at the point of death; please come and*

lay Your hands on her, that she **may get well** (sozo) and live." Mark 5:23

Mark's Gospel relates that Jairus asked for salvation in the form of healing for his daughter. Luke reveals that Jesus also used this word in response to Jairus. Jesus told Jairus that his daughter would be _saved, delivered, set free, made whole, and made well_ if he _believed_. In this case, the translators chose _made well_.

But when Jesus heard this, He answered him, "Do not be afraid any longer; only believe, and she **shall be made well** (sozo)." Luke 8:50

The story reveals that Christ's _salvation_ for Jairus' daughter was her resurrection from the dead rather than a simple healing. She had died before Christ arrived to heal her. Obviously, _sozo_ may include resurrections as well as healing and deliverance. These two places bring the total to eleven places where some form of _healing_ is revealed as _salvation_. It is noteworthy that Christ also tells Jairus to _believe and she will be made well_. Faith again brings _salvation_ in the form of healing.

The Healing of the Blind Beggar Bartimaeus

The healing of the blind man Bartimaeus also reveals _salvation as healing_ in two of the gospels. Mark writes:

And Jesus said to him, "Go your way; your faith **has made you well** (sozo)." And immediately he _regained his sight and began following Him on the road. Mark 10:52_

Faith is also indicated as the reason that Bartimaeus was able to receive salvation in the form of healing. Luke writes of the same event of healing and records the identical words of Christ to Bartimaeus:

And Jesus said to him, "Receive your sight; your faith **has made you well** (sozo)." Luke 18:42

Salvation came to Bartimaeus in the form of healing of his blindness. Christ says in both verses that _faith_ releases _salvation_ in the form of _healing_. This brings our total to thirteen places in the New Testament where a form of _sozo_ is used in reference to healing.

The Man with a Legion of Demons
The fourteenth account where a form of the word _sozo_ is used in reference to healing is the man with Legion. The word _Legion_ is a Roman military term. A Roman legion was normally about 6000 soldiers. So what is strongly implied in this passage is that this man was insane because he had 6000 demons. The story relates that Christ delivers this man from a great number of demons. _Salvation_ for this insane man included _deliverance from demons_ that can cause conditions of _insanity._

And those who had seen it reported to them how the man who was demon-possessed **had been made well** (sozo). Luke 8:36

306

Healing is an Aspect of Salvation

The Greek word in this passage could have been translated _delivered, made whole,_ or _set free_ rather than _made well._ All these phrases would be appropriate. This man was _healed_ because he experienced _salvation_ in the _form of deliverance from evil spirits._

The Cleansing of Ten Lepers

In a conversation with one of the ten lepers who were cleansed from leprosy, Christ says this:

> _And He said to him, "Rise, and go your way; your faith **has made you well** (sozo)." Luke 17:19_

Cleansing from _an infectious disease_ is also a form of _salvation._ This brings the total to fifteen uses of _sozo_ in reference to some form of healing.

Peter Healed the Lame Man at the Temple

Luke's Gospel relates through Peter's words that the lame man who Peter healed at the temple experienced salvation in the form of healing. In Peter's explanation to the critical leaders of Israel, he describes the healing using a form of _sozo._

> _...if we are on trial today for a benefit done to a sick man, as to how this man **has been made well** (sozo)... Acts 4:9_

Peter earlier explained the healing to the observers much like Christ does in some of the passages. Peter said that _faith_ in the name of Jesus Christ had _strengthened_ and given this man _perfect health._

> *And on the basis of **faith** in His name, it is the name of Jesus which has **strengthened** this man whom you see and know; and the **faith** which comes through Him has given him this **perfect health** in the presence of you all. Acts 3:16*

This reads much like Christ's statement, *"your faith has made you well"* found many times in the Gospels. In fact, the statement of Peter contains exactly the same ideas. Peter apparently had learned this lesson from Christ and understood exactly what had caused this healing. There was no mystery here to Peter. This was the sixteenth use of a form of *sozo* in a passage that reveals a healing.

Paul Heals the Lame Man in Lystra
Luke also tells us that another lame man in Lystra experienced salvation in the form of healing. In this case, Paul, rather than Peter, was involved in the healing of this man.

> *This man was listening to Paul as he spoke, who, when he had fixed his gaze upon him, and had seen that he had faith **to be made well** (sozo)... Acts 14:9*

Noteworthy is the reference again to *faith*. This is the seventeenth use of a form of *sozo* in a passage that involves a healing.

Healing is an Aspect of Salvation

General Encouragement

The book of James also has a verse that reveals salvation in the form of healing. It also points to faith as the condition for receiving healing. James reveals:

> _...and the prayer offered in faith **will restore** (sozo) the one who is sick, and the Lord will raise him up, and if he has committed sins, they will be forgiven him...James 5:15_

This is the eighteenth and final use of a form of _sozo_ in the New Testament in passages that concern healing.

Powerful Implications of Healing as Salvation

The fact that the New Testament writers repeatedly used forms of the word _sozo_ in healing passages has strong implications for a biblical theology of healing. As discussed earlier in this book, often healing is treated in a different fashion than other aspects of salvation. These are some of the implications:

- **Salvation in All Forms Because of the Cross**

Some have wanted, for doctrinal reasons, to disconnect healing from salvation by disconnecting healing from the cross. However, this is impossible to do if the New Testament is to be taken seriously in the formation of a theology of healing. Matthew connects healing and deliverance in the ministry of Christ with the prophecy of Isaiah which predicts the atonement of Christ at Calvary.

> _And when evening had come, they brought to Him many who were demon-possessed; and He cast out_

the spirits with a word, and healed all who were ill in order that what was spoken through Isaiah the prophet might be fulfilled, saying, "HE HIMSELF TOOK OUR INFIRMITIES, AND CARRIED AWAY OUR DISEASES." Matthew 8:16-17

Study of this quotation from Isaiah, Chapter 53 should forever remove any doubt that healing was purchased by Christ at the cross. The rest of this chapter is quoted repeatedly throughout the New Testament. Isaiah's prophecy describes what Christ would accomplish from the Father's perspective. The New Testament authors unquestionably recognize Isaiah, Chapter 53 as describing the effect of the sacrifice of the coming Christ. For example, like Matthew, the apostle Peter describes the sacrifice of Jesus Christ by quoting from Isaiah, Chapter 53. Peter writes *for by His wounds you were healed.* Peter obviously recognized that Isaiah Chapter 53 predicted the work of Christ on the cross and makes mention of healing as well.

...and He Himself bore our sins in His body on the cross, that we might die to sin and live to righteousness; for by His wounds you were healed. 1 Peter 2:24

Three witnesses have spoken on this matter. Isaiah, Matthew and Peter have testified that the cross purchases salvation in the form of healing. Healing is in the atonement of Christ. The cross where Christ died for the forgiveness of sins and regeneration also purchases healing and deliverance from evil spirits. The same truths that apply to the forgiveness of sins and regeneration also apply to healing and deliverance.

The Father's Will for Salvation in All Forms

If forgiveness of sins and regeneration are _already settled_ as the Father's will, then healing and deliverance are _already settled_ as well. If the Father _always_ wants people saved from sin, then He _always_ wants people delivered from demons. If the Father _always_ wants to forgive the sins of the repentant, then He _always_ wants to heal those who meet His conditions for healing. The Father's will is _settled_ and _never changes_ in matters of salvation in all its forms. The only issue is meeting the Father's conditions to receive the Lord Jesus Christ as Savior, Healer or Deliverer.

• Faith for Salvation-Faith for Healing

If faith in Christ is a condition of receiving salvation in the form of forgiveness of sins, then it is also a condition of healing and deliverance. If faith is required for salvation and healing, then the same truths apply. For instance, salvation in the form of forgiveness of sins, regeneration, and eternal life comes on the basis of faith in Jesus Christ as Savior. In like manner, salvation in the form of healing comes because of faith in Jesus Christ as Healer.

The vast majority of people can be healed by a simple response of faith in Christ as their Healer after they settle in their hearts that the Father wants them well. When these last doubts about the will of the Father are gone, then simple but overcoming faith will be present. A very few, who seem to have legitimate faith, need to resolve other issues that are blocking the grace of God to them.

However, the difficulty of a few in receiving healing does not change the fact of the Father wanting them whole.

The Predictability of Healing

Most believers who are knowledgeable of the Bible would not accept that someone being *born again* is unpredictable. They would say that being *born again* is dependent upon someone *hearing the Good News* about Jesus Christ as Lord and Savior in an understandable way. Then, after hearing the Good News (the gospel), a *person must respond in faith* and *accept Jesus Christ as Lord and Savior.* (Of course, repentance is necessary in accepting Christ as Lord.) In other words, most believers that are knowledgeable of the Bible would say that it is *always* the Father's will for persons to be *born again* when they meet the conditions. Likewise, healing is dependent upon *hearing the Good News* about *Jesus as Healer* in an understandable way. Then responding in *faith* to that message by receiving Christ as their *Healer.* Therefore, healing becomes predictable and reliable when and where the gospel is boldly preached, revealing Christ as Healer and unbiblical doctrines producing doubts about healing are assaulted and rejected.

• The Timing of Healing

Some seem to be *waiting for a sovereign act* of God for healing. This is a misunderstanding of the Father's will for healing. This *waiting* for the Father *to do something* that the New Testament declares as *already done* is counterproductive. This misunderstanding may actually block healing.

Healing is an Aspect of Salvation

It is _already_ the Father's will for healing. Salvation from sin is _already_ the Father's will. The timing of salvation from sin is _now_. No one would foolishly tell someone seeking Christ for forgiveness that maybe it is not time for them to be saved. Obviously, the timing of forgiveness is when a decision is made for Christ. The proper timing is _as soon as possible._ The Divine side of the equation is complete. Christ has died for their sins. _It is finished!_ Only the human side of the equation of salvation needs to be completed. In other words, the issue is never the Father's timing but the person's decision to believe in Christ as their personal Savior. Consider Paul's words concerning the timing of salvation:

> _And working together with Him, we also urge you not to receive the grace of God in vain-- for He says, "AT THE ACCEPTABLE TIME I LISTENED TO YOU, AND ON THE DAY OF SALVATION I HELPED YOU"; behold, **now** is "THE ACCEPTABLE TIME," behold, **now** is THE DAY OF SALVATION "-- 2 Corinthians 6:1-2_

Forgiveness of sins has _already_ been purchased at Calvary. Forgiveness is _available_ when faith in Christ as Savior arises in the heart of a believer. _Now is the acceptable time_ for forgiveness. _Now_ is the time to believe.

Likewise, healing has _already_ been purchased at Calvary. Healing is _available_ when faith in Christ as Healer arises in the heart of a person. _Now is the acceptable time for healing._ These same truths apply to deliverance from evil spirits. *Now is the acceptable time for deliverance. Now* is the time to believe.

Those seeking healing are not trying to convince the Father to heal them. The Father has already healed them in Christ. They must simply receive Christ as Healer *just like* they received Christ as Savior. They must believe in Christ as their Healer and stand in His truth *until* the full manifestation of healing occurs. Christ remains their Healer *regardless of their experience.* However, overcoming faith in Christ as Healer will release the power of the Holy Spirit to *change their experience.*

~15~

Questions and Answers

If someone has the gift of healing, why don't they go and empty out the hospitals?

If healing were entirely in the control of the person who has the gift, then this would be possible. However, the New Testament reveals that healing *nearly always* involves the faith of the person being prayed for or the faith of a relative or friend. While there are a few noteworthy exceptions in the ministry of Christ worth considering, the vast majority of biblical healings reveal that someone, in addition to Christ, had faith for the healing. As the ministry of Christ is analyzed, there seem to be four clear categories of the kinds of persons Christ healed. There are also two categories of persons not healed in Christ's ministry. These categories seem to explain why a person with the gift of healing cannot empty out a hospital. *Here are the four categories of those who were healed:*

There were those who came to Christ on their own and were healed. Their faith was evident by their behavior because they came to Christ for healing. Thousands of people seemed to receive their healing this way. Most often, these people received healing in Christ's mass healing events. However, some of the specific healings in Christ's ministry also fit this category, such as healing of the woman with the issue of blood[1]. Christ often

---

1. Matthew 9:20-22, Mark 5:25-34, Luke 8:43-48

responded to these people by saying *your faith has healed you.* This category seems to cover the great majority of Christ's healings and seems to be the most ordinary way to conduct healing ministry.

There were those who were brought by someone else to Christ and were healed. In these cases, the faith of someone else was evident by their behavior. Again, thousands of people seemed to receive their healing in this way, and often received healing in Christ's mass healing events. A few specific examples also fit this category, such as the man whose friends lowered him through the roof to Jesus. The account says that Jesus, *seeing their faith,* healed this man[2]. Together categories 1 and 2 seem to cover the vast majority of healings in Christ's ministry.

There were those in need of healing who could not come, but someone else -- a friend or relative -- sought for Christ to come to the needy person. There are a handful of recorded examples in the Gospels of Christ regarding this type of healing. Again, the faith of another person who cared about the sick or injured person was involved in the healing. Their faith was revealed by their effort to get Christ to come to the person in need. The healing of the Centurion's servant[3] and the healing of the Syrophenian woman's daughter[4] are situations that fit this category. In each of these two situations, Christ gives credit for the healing to the faith of the relative or friend. While this is not an extraordinary way to heal, it is still a much less frequent way that Christ healed the sick.

There were those who did not come at all and Christ seemed to seek them out for healing. There seem to be *only a very few*

2. Matthew 9:1-8, Mark 2:1-12, Luke 5:17-26
3. Matthew 8:5-13
4. Matthew 15:21-28

examples of this among the thousands of healings and miracles in the ministry of Christ. These healings are extraordinary, and it is important that healing theology acknowledges that they are extraordinary. It seems practical and prudent that the theological foundation for healing be based on the ordinary rather than the extraordinary. One of these examples is found in the Gospel of John, Chapter 5. The man at the pool at Bethesda had been sick thirty-eight years and Christ initiated the events of this man's healing. In fact, even after the man was healed, he did not know who had healed him. In this case, it appears that Christ purposely went to the pool in Jerusalem where there were a great number of sick and injured people. It is possible that Christ may have been looking for someone whom He could heal in order to get all the suffering people at this pool to believe in Him as their Healer. After healing this man, it is likely that the good news about this healing reached the ears of many that were seeking healing at Bethesda's pool. It is also possible that many of them sought out healing from Christ in the weeks and months to follow. In this case, Christ was able to use His own faith to produce the healing of this man. Christ seemed to catch this man completely by surprise. A second example in the ministry of Christ is the resurrection of the widow's son found in Luke 7:11-18. In this account, it appears that Christ has again surprised everyone with this miracle. There is no chance of anyone responding either negatively or positively to Christ in this matter. In these two cases, it appears that Christ's own faith is enough to accomplish the work of the Father, as long as He does not encounter unbelief and doubt among the people He is seeking to serve. Perhaps surprising someone avoids an unbelieving response. Emptying a hospital would require this type of extraordinary healing repeatedly. Considering Christ's limitations in His own hometown, not even He would be able to accomplish this. This would be similar to the situation at the pool at Bethesda. The afflicted people at this pool were not seeking Christ as Healer, and He was limited in the help that He could offer. Only this man was healed at that particular time. The vast majority of people in hospitals are not seeking Christ for healing. This is much like the pool at Bethesda. The people at this pool in that story were not seeking healing from Christ. Christ only healed the one man. Therefore, any help that a person with healing gifts could offer in a secular hospital under normal conditions would be limited. However, individuals within that hospital setting could be healed under the right conditions of faith.

The other two categories that must be considered are those who were *not healed* in Christ's ministry.

Some were not healed because they did not come to Christ because they did not hear about Him healing. The majority of those who remained ill or injured in Israel were those who did not come to be healed. They did not come simply because they did not hear the Good News that Christ is Healer. Of course, the same problem remains today. The Gospel is often preached without acknowledging Christ as Healer. Consequently, many Christian people do not respond in faith to Christ, the Healer and struggle on with sickness and injury when healing is available.

Some who heard about Christ healing people responded in unbelief, did not come and were not healed. In Christ's own hometown, the people responded in unbelief to Him, and Christ was unable to do much to help the sick and injured there. The implication of unbelief is present in many passages. Christ's critics and persecutors among the religious leaders were certainly unbelieving. Very probably some of these critics and their families were in need of healing but did not come because of unbelief. Although Christ was present and healing was available, most of them were not healed. Today, critics of healing ministry are likely to be in the same situation. Their criticism and unbelief will prevent them from seeking a Christian person with the gift of healing in operation.

Doesn't a strong emphasis on faith condemn those who are struggling with sickness?

No. It should not condemn anyone. Anyone can obtain faith for healing. Christ Himself put great emphasis on faith in matters of healing. Therefore, anyone wishing to emulate the Savior's supernatural ministry must also teach as He taught. In many of the accounts of His healings and miracles, Christ took the opportunity to comment or teach about faith.

Misunderstandings concerning the nature of faith are what create condemnation. Some have taught faith as if it were a static, unchanging thing. In those situations, they have improperly taught that either you have faith or you do not have it. However, true faith constantly changes. Faith has to do with our active reliance upon Christ. Therefore, faith can grow or decrease in strength.

Faith is affected by our understanding of the Father's will. Faith is affected by our theology. Faith is affected by doubts. Faith is affected by the clarity of our revelation of the love of God. Therefore, prayer and diligent Bible study can affect faith as long as we allow the Holy Spirit to use these means to adjust us.

Faith for healing often comes to an individual after hearing a bold proclamation of Jesus Christ as Healer. In other words, faith can be released. Faith is not static, but a dynamic reliance upon a faithful Healer. While a person may have been weak in faith yesterday, they may have their faith released today by a faithful presentation of the Gospel. While they may be struggling today, the destruction of a theological doubt, a mental stronghold, can release a brand new experience of healing tomorrow. No one should ever allow the enemy to condemn them as they seek to know Christ as their Healer. The enemy wants them to give up. However, the Father is on their side and will work with them until they are healed.

What about people who have strong faith in Christ as Healer and have not been healed?

This is a difficult question to answer. It is difficult because the question has an answer that is troublesome to some and offensive to others. The answer can make it seem as if those who are doing healing ministry are hard-hearted and insensitive to the struggles and suffering of some of God's people. The answer can produce defensiveness and reactions of loyalty in those who have genuine compassion for those that are struggling. However, the question must be addressed clearly if theological doubts are going to be completely removed from God's people on the matter of healing and help offered to these struggling believers. The question itself has several important hidden assumptions that need to be addressed.

First, the question seems to indicate that the unhealed person's faith was unmistakable. However, experience has revealed that these situations are often not what they seem on the surface. Often the very real and *strong faith* of these struggling people is mixed with significant theological doubts and misunderstandings of healing. These doubts can only be discerned and revealed by in-depth counseling with these persons. Fortunately, today there are more Christians being equipped to deal with these doubts biblically. Many times, biblical counseling and working through a sick person's doubts will result in their healing. Christ points out the relationship between *faith* and *doubt* in Mark's Gospel.

Questions and Answers

*Truly I say to you, whoever says to this mountain, 'Be taken up and cast into the sea,' **and does not doubt in his heart**, but **believes** that what he says is going to happen, it shall be granted him. Mark 11:23*

This is encouraging. Those who believe that they have faith in Christ as Healer and have not yet received healing need only to seek to remove their doubts. Many times this is the case of those who have not received. They have faith in Christ but their remaining doubts prohibit their receiving.

Secondly, the question also assumes something that cannot be assumed. The question assumes that we can know if another person has faith. Faith is an issue of the heart. No one knows his or her own heart much less the heart of another person. Love, compassion and loyalty sometimes makes us want to assume something about a person that we love that may not be entirely true and cannot be known for sure about another person or even ourselves. It is difficult to be objective about matters that involve us so personally.

Likewise, we are likely to confuse hope, sincerity and possibly even desperation with faith. We are likely to assume that some actions reveal faith such as lengthy passionate prayer and fasting. However, none of these things are faith. They are good works that may or may not be inspired by faith in Christ. Fear and desperation rather than faith may inspire these good works.

Thirdly, the question also presupposes that it is possible to have faith for healing and not be healed. This assumes that the Father's promises of healing, numerous as they may be, are not reliable as God's promises are in other matters. It assumes that the Father is a respecter of persons, doing for one person what He will not for another although the same conditions were met. All of these assumptions are decidedly unscriptural and do weaken faith in Christ as Healer. In other words, the assumption that it is possible to have faith for healing and not be healed is full of doubt itself. The real doubts that this unscriptural idea produces could be the reason that healing has not yet come. God is *always* faithful to fulfill all His promises when the conditions are met.

Fourth, this question invites the blame game. This makes it an unhealthy question. It balances the righteousness of the unhealed person against the righteousness of God. Either we must blame the unhealed person or we must subtly blame God for not fulfilling His promises. Those who blame God and justify the unhealed person often are blind to their behavior. They generally cannot see that they are blaming God and presenting Him as mysterious, unpredictable and unreliable in the matter of healing. This, of course, creates future doubts for everyone affected by this presentation of God. Blaming anyone -- God or the unhealed person -- is unproductive for the Kingdom of God. Let us affirm that God is faithful to His promises and patiently work with unhealed people to receive His grace without resorting to the *blame game*.

What about Job? Doesn't the Book of Job demonstrate that God is not always willing to heal?

No. The book of Job does not demonstrate that God is not always willing to heal. We must remind the reader that the Old Testament revelation of God is incomplete. Christ alone completely reveals the Father's will. This is particularly true concerning healing. Basing a theology of healing on Job rather than Jesus Christ will certainly cause confusion. Besides these things, the Book of Job is often misunderstood. However, the Book of Job does demonstrate a number of important things that are largely ignored by complex theology.

Questions and Answers

First, *Satan afflicted Job with sickness, not God.* Often complex doctrine wants to over-emphasize that God initiated the conversation with Satan and gave permission to Satan before he could touch Job. This overemphasis creates a *leap-in-logic* that creates serious theological doubts. This *leap-in-logic* says this:

> **When God allows something to occur, then it is His will for that thing to happen. This is simply because God already knows what the result will be when He allows something to occur. In other words, if God does not prevent something or intervene in the process, then what is happening must be God's will.**

This *leap-in-logic* in effect reverses the stated truth of Scripture that Satan made Job ill. It creates a doctrinal viewpoint that states that God wanted and made Job sick. The Scripture does not say this. This twisted logic is imposed on Scripture and that produces doubts. Just because God allows something to occur does not mean that it is His will. God's foreknowledge does not mean that all things happen according to God's will. All the things that occur in the earth are clearly not God's will. If all things that occur were God's will, then all the sin, injustices, losses, tragedies, and pain of the world would then become God's will. This is not so. This is a *demonic view of God* presented by popular but extreme theologies and western culture. These theologies present God as if He were responsible for and doing all the destructive works of the devil. In contrast, the Bible declares that the devil, demonic activity and the sinfulness of humanity are the actual causes of the sad condition of the world. God, our Father, is not the cause of the *brokenness* of the world. Jesus Christ perfectly reveals the Father's will in restoration and healing of brokenness. Christ destroys the destructive works of the devil and brings restoration, recovery and healing to all who come to Him. Christ *never* causes anyone to be sick or injured. This expresses the true will of God, our Father and is Good News. The complex theological view that God is the cause of the sad condition of the world and the suffering of humanity is not Good News and is therefore wrong.

Secondly, *God did heal Job*. Somehow, this fact escapes most people who know about Job. In fact, Job lived to be 140 years old. The last chapter of the book indicates that Job was greatly blessed by God after his sickness and experienced a *double restoration* of all the things that he had lost at the hands of the devil. The account reveals that Satan robbed, killed, destroyed and afflicted, but God healed, delivered and restored. Complex theology confuses these simple biblical facts.

Furthermore, if someone believes that they are experiencing a mysterious dealing from God like Job's involving sickness, then they should expect that the final result would be healing and health, not further sickness or death. When a person dies without healing, then it should be clear to others that the sick person was *not* experiencing a *Job-like* dealing from God or they would have eventually recovered.

Thirdly, Job's three religious friends played *the blame game* with him and were wrong in their conclusions of why Job was sick. Job was wrong also in his conclusions of why he was sick. The tendency of Job's friends was to blame Job. In kind of a defensive reaction, Job eventually began to blame God. No one ever seemed to blame the real source of Job's condition, which was the devil. Eventually, in the last chapter of the Book of Job, God corrected the three friends who had blamed Job. God also corrected Job for blaming Him.

The whole painful and difficult circumstance brought out some issues that needed dealing with in Job's life. A young man, Elihu, who had been silent throughout *the blame game* debate between Job and his three friends finally spoke up and corrected Job and his three friends for playing *the blame game.*

> *Then these three men ceased answering Job, because he was righteous in his own eyes. But the anger of Elihu...burned; against Job his anger burned, because he justified himself before God. And his anger burned against his three friends because they had found no answer, and yet had condemned Job. Job 32:1-3*

In other words, Elihu was angry with Job and his three friends. They were all wrong. Job has complained repeatedly that he has done nothing wrong. He had repeatedly declared his righteousness. Job went so far as to blame God (not the devil) for his problems. Job's three friends had been trying to make an accusation against him for dozens of chapters to explain why these things have happened. Finally, the young man, Elihu, begins to put things into a proper order. Elihu spends a few chapters explaining why Job cannot proclaim that he is innocent and righteous and why Job cannot blame God for his predicament. For instance, Elihu sums up and corrects Job's attitude expressed in *the blame game* that he has been playing with his religious friends.

> *"For Job has said, 'I am righteous, But God has taken away my right; Should I lie concerning my right? My wound is incurable, though I am without transgression.' ... Job 34:5-6*

Elihu continues his correction of Job and his friends a few verses later.

> *For he (Job) has said, 'It profits a man nothing When he is pleased with God.' Therefore, listen to me, you men of*

understanding. Far be it from God to do wickedness, And from the Almighty to do wrong. Job 34:9-10

Elihu understands that when a man justifies himself, he subtly blames God for his situation. When a man declares his lack of fault in a situation, then his tendency will be to subtly argue that God did not do what He said He would do. Often the accusation against God is cloaked in religiosity but is still there. God apparently agrees with Elihu's assessment of the situation and begins to correct Job in similar fashion in Chapter 38. This leads to Job's repentance from self-righteousness and his healing and restoration. Therefore, one of the Book of Job's best lessons is that *the blame game* should be avoided. Justifying yourself or justifying another person in the matter of sickness and healing enters *the blame game* and subtly blames God. It is better to continue to seek the Healer than to begin to declare that there is no fault in the one seeking healing. It is better to say that we are doing all that we know to do but there may be more to learn. After the untimely death of a loved one from sickness, there is no need to play *the blame game* either. The results of *the blame game* are harmful to others seeking healing because they produce serious doubts about God's faithfulness.

You say that Christ reveals that it is the Father's will to always heal. Doesn't Paul's thorn in the flesh reveal that God was not willing to heal Paul?

Poor teaching about Paul's *thorn in the flesh* has created doubts in the minds of many people. These doubts have been sufficient to block healing for many people. Therefore, it is necessary to thoroughly analyze the passage from which these ideas that produce doubt come. The primary verse in question is found in Paul's Second letter to the Corinthians. This verse reads:

And because of the surpassing greatness of the revelations, for this reason, to keep me from exalting myself, there was given me a thorn in the flesh, a messenger of Satan to buffet me-- to keep me from exalting myself! 2 Corinthians 12:7

These are the questions that will be considered in analysis of this verse:

- _What is the context of the verse?_
- _What does the verse actually say that the thorn is?_
- _What does the Greek word that is translated "thorn" reveal?_

Hopefully after these questions are answered honestly, then a good interpretation of the verse will be apparent. Our first consideration, therefore, is the context of the verse.

The context of these verses is revealing. At the end of the previous chapter, Paul is relating all the suffering, dangers, beatings, and imprisonment that he endured for the sake of the Gospel. He does not mention sickness. In that context in chapter 11, Paul speaks of being _weak_ but certainly not as a reference to sickness but as a reference to the difficulties that he endured.

At the beginning of chapter 12, Paul begins to explain that he had special revelations of Paradise, of the third heaven. Then he begins to speak of a thorn in the flesh given to keep him from _exalting himself_ as a result of the _surpassing revelations_ of the _third heaven, paradise. Therefore, by implication, a thorn in the flesh is given when someone has special surpassing revelation from God._ An important truth emerges that should help most people's faith:

Most people, therefore, would not qualify for a thorn in the flesh no matter what the thorn may be simply because they are not having surpassing revelations of paradise like Paul describes.

Paul says that he asked the Lord three times to remove the thorn but the Lord answered that His grace was sufficient for Paul and that _power was made perfect in weakness._ The word for _weakness_ is again used. There are a number of Greek words used in the New Testament used exclusively for sickness. This word is not one of them. It was also used a few verses earlier in the previous passage in a context that has to do with persecution. It is probable that Paul is using _weakness_ again in this way. In fact, a verse in the next chapter seems to indicate this strongly. Both words, _power_ and _weakness,_ are also used in this verse. In this verse, Paul says:

For indeed He (Christ) was crucified because of weakness, yet He lives because of the power of God. For we also are weak in Him, yet we shall live with Him because of the power of God directed toward you.
2 Corinthians 13:4

Clearly, in this context, Paul is not saying that _weakness_ is sickness. In fact, Paul says that Christ was crucified because of _weakness._ It puts the term _weakness_ into the context of what unbelieving people were able to do to Christ. They were able to persecute Him to the point of crucifixion. Paul uses the word in the same way. Paul's _weakness_ was _the suffering that he had to endure at the hands of enemies._

In addition, the ordinary words exclusively used for sickness in other passages do not appear anywhere in the context. Additionally, just a few verses after writing about the _thorn_ Paul writes that the _signs of the apostle_ were present in his ministry. He mentions *signs, wonders and miracles.* It seems rather unlikely that Paul would tell his readers about his own sickness and then a few verses later tell about his ability to do miracles. The context reveals that this *weakness,* the *thorn in the flesh,* must be something other than a sickness or a medical condition of some type.

- *What does the verse actually say that the thorn is?*

The verse actually does reveal what the *thorn* is. Paul says that the *thorn* is *a messenger of Satan.* The Greek word that is translated *messenger* is the same word that is often transliterated as *angel* elsewhere in the New Testament. Paul tells us that the thorn in the flesh is *an angel of Satan.* It is quite a *leap-of-logic* to say that this is sickness. Paul is describing a fallen angel as his thorn in the flesh. Since Paul tells us through the context of all the persecutions he received, a more reasonable interpretation would be that Paul was asking the Lord to stop the actions of a fallen angel who stirred up persecution against Paul wherever he went. In the same way that the devil stirred up trouble leading to the crucifixion of Christ, Paul was suffering trouble caused by this fallen angel. This seems to be validated by further study of the words used in this context.

- *What does the Greek word that is translated "thorn" reveal?*

The use of this Greek word reveals a great deal. The Greek word that is translated *thorn* is *skolop.* This Greek word only appears in the New Testament in this verse. However, this Greek word appears three times in the Septuagint, the ancient Greek translation of the Old Testament. A great deal of evidence exists that suggests that Paul and other First Century preachers used the Septuagint to preach from throughout the ancient world. Therefore, it is probable that the apostle Paul was very familiar with how *skolop* was used in this ancient version of the Old Testament.

Skolop is found in three passages in the Septuagint; Numbers 33:55, Ezekiel 28:24 and Hosea 2:6. In Numbers, this word is used in reference to the enemies of Israel.

> *But if you do not drive out the inhabitants of the land from before you, then it shall come about that those whom you let remain of them will become as pricks in your eyes and as thorns (skolop) in your sides, and they shall trouble you in the land in which you live.*
> *Numbers 33:55*

This use of *skolop* above seems to support the interpretation that suggests that Paul's thorn in the flesh had to do with persecution from enemies stirred up by a fallen angel. The passage above does not support the idea that sickness was in some way involved.

The second place where *skolop* is used is found in the Book of Ezekiel. In the context of this verse, God is declaring that Sidon and other enemies will no longer be a *thorn* in Israel's side. This usage seems to support the idea that the *thorn* has to do with enemies rather than sickness.

> *And there will be no more for the house of Israel a prickling brier or a painful thorn (skolop) from any round about them who scorned them; then they will know that I am the Lord GOD. Ezekiel 28:24*

In Hosea, the use of this word is not as clear as the previous two uses. The verse simply says that God will prevent His people from going after false lovers by a wall of thorns.

> *Therefore, behold, I will hedge up her way with thorns,(skolop) And I will build a wall against her so that she cannot find her paths. Hosea 2:6*

This particular use does not reveal anything else to help except that the verse does not reveal *skolop* as having a connection to sickness. None of the three uses of this word in the Greek Old Testament relate to sickness and two seem to be clearly related to difficulties with enemies.

In summary, a close analysis of this verse does not reveal that Paul had a sickness or injury. In fact, the verse itself reveals that an *angel of Satan* was the problem and the context reveals that *difficulties from enemies is the weakness* that Paul asks the Lord to remove. Suggestions from other verses that Paul had eye problems, or other conditions such as speech difficulties, are often built upon the assumptions that Paul's thorn in the flesh was a medical condition. However, the biblical foundation for these speculations and theological doubts is very weak. It is extremely unlikely that Paul's thorn in the flesh was a medical condition. However, we cannot conclusively say that Paul never had a medical condition to deal with. What we can conclude, however, is that Paul could receive healing like any other believer. Therefore, Paul does not provide an example of someone that God was not willing to heal.

Is it possible that the power of suggestion is the cause of what appears to be supernatural Christian healing?

Assuming this would be placing a great deal of undeserved faith in the power of suggestion rather in what the Bible reveals about healing. There is no doubt that positive thinking and emotions have a supportive effect on the physical body's ability to heal itself just as negative thinking and emotions have a destructive effect. Research has shown this is true as well as that which has been described as *the placebo effect*. Improvement of medical conditions have been shown when someone simply *believes* that a medication or treatment is helping them even if the "medication" is really a *placebo* that is not really affecting their condition. Belief seems to reinforce the body's limited ability to heal itself even if that belief is not placed in Christ as Healer. For a number of important spiritual reasons we do not recommend hypnosis but acknowledge that hypnosis does seem to help some people with pain and addictive and destructive habits. What hypnosis and the placebo effect are able to accomplish are the limitations of what the power of suggestion is actually able to do. *If healing ministry is being accomplished by the power of suggestion then why don't we see secular experts on suggestion healing the seriously ill and seriously injured?* We do not see hypno-therapists, psychologists, and psychiatrists healing seriously ill or injured people physically or regularly. On the other hand, these limitations are removed when biblical healing is considered. Multitudes of seriously ill or injured people worldwide are being healed each year through faith in the name of Jesus Christ. Most of these healings are instantaneous and cannot be explained by the body's natural limited capacity to heal itself. Additionally, some that are unable to believe because they are so seriously ill or injured are being healed because someone else prayed and believed for them. The power of suggestion could not have played at part at all in many healings like these.

Is all supernatural healing from God?

No. Supernatural healing that comes from any source that does not acknowledge Jesus Christ as Savior, Lord, Deliverer and Healer is not from God. The occult, other world religions and new age sources all would fit into this category. The deceptive power behind these religions is the god of this world, Satan. The devil will do things through his sincere but mistaken servants that deceptively appear to be good. Since demonic activity is the cause of much sickness, Satan simply removes the sickness temporarily to deceive the unwary. Satan does these things to keep people bound by false religions and beliefs that will not save them eternally.

Are manifestations necessary for healing ministry?

No. Faith in Christ as Healer is all that is necessary for healing. Healing can and often does occur without anyone feeling anything. However, manifestations allow the believer and the minister of healing to know that healing has taken place. Manifestations of various types, such as heat or electricity (strong tingling) in the hands of the one praying or in the area of the body needing healing, are an ordinary way that the Holy Spirit communicates with us. Other manifestations are possible but in our experience are not as common. Manifestations such as falling down (commonly called being *slain in the Spirit*) or *holy laughter* are legitimate expressions of the work of the Holy Spirit at times. However, these manifestations can be counterproductive to mass healing ministry if too many people adjust psychologically to performing these particular manifestations when they feel the presence of the Holy Spirit. Often they will fall down *before* they are healed or be unable to cooperate with the healing minister if they lose control laughing. When these things happen, often people that could have been healed are not.

Can anyone heal the sick? What if I don't have the gift of healing?

Yes. Anyone who is a true believer in Jesus Christ can heal the sick since Christ the Healer is living within them. Some believers might be better equipped and spiritually gifted. Some believers might have more faith than others. Some believers might have more experience. Some believers might have better overall or ongoing results but anyone who believes can heal the sick. Additionally, Paul records in 1 Corinthians 14:1 that we should *desire earnestly spiritual gifts*. This strongly suggests that we can obtain gifts from God that we don't presently have. Paul reveals in Romans 1:11, 2 Timothy 1:6, and 1 Timothy 4:14 that spiritual gifts can be imparted from a gifted person to someone who is not gifted previously. Ephesians 4:11-12 says that believers are *to be equipped for ministry*. So we can expect to become increasingly more gifted than we are presently.

Is deliverance ministry necessary for healing ministry?

Yes and no. If a servant of God is going to have consistent results in healing the sick, they must understand and be able to practice deliverance ministry. This is simply because some of the sick, injured, or disabled people that they encounter are being afflicted by demons. About one-quarter of the healings in Christ's ministry appear to involve deliverance from evil spirits. The servant of God must work through their theological doubts concerning deliverance ministry if they are going to have consistent results in healing ministry. However, since the majority of medical conditions are not being caused by demonic activity, it is possible to accomplish a great deal of healing without practicing and understanding or even believing in deliverance.

Is the inner healing of the emotions needed before physical healing can be obtained?

No. We must defer to Christ's example. Nowhere in the Gospels do we see Christ making the healing of emotions a prerequisite for physical healing. There is no doubt that Christ does heal the brokenhearted but there does not seem to be a clear scriptural connection that would make healing of the emotions a primary concern before healing of the physical body of sick or injured persons. This idea that inner emotional healing must occur first is not biblical and may be a reflection of the affect of the beliefs of modern psychology on the modern Church. However, deliverance from evil spirits could be a prerequisite for physical healing and emotional healing since some physical sickness and emotional problems are a result of the destructive work of demons.

Is there any opposition between Divine healing and medical care?

No. The body itself reveals that it is God's will to heal. God has so designed the body that it has its own limited ability to heal itself. When that innate power to heal requires assistance through medicine, herbs, diet, rest or any other natural means, it is within the will of God to obtain that help. We encourage anyone sick or injured to seek all the natural help that they need in the process of believing in Christ as Healer. Christ is not limited to the natural or to the supernatural. Christ may use a doctor and a minister of healing together to bring wholeness. The only caution that should be given is where medical care crosses over into supernatural methodology. When medical caregivers begin to use occultic or new age techniques or techniques borrowed from other religions such as Buddhism or Hinduism, this kind of "medical care" should be rejected.

What is the relationship between lifestyle and healing?

Obviously, there is a relationship between lifestyle and sickness. One can live in such a way to break down their health. However, lifestyle and healing have a different relationship. Healing can be received because of faith in Christ no matter what the previous lifestyle has been. Forgiveness of sins must be acknowledged as a foundation for the entirety of what God does. However, conscience also plays a part in the matter of faith. If one lives a lifestyle that produces sickness in them, then a guilty conscience makes it more difficult to believe for healing. Likewise, if a person lives a righteous lifestyle, seeing their life and body as stewardship from God, then the conscience is clear and healing is much easier to receive. Therefore, it is generally easier for people who live righteously to receive healing when they need it. This is not because they deserve healing but simply because their conscience is clearer. Healing is a matter of the unmerited favor of God. It is a matter of mercy and grace and cannot be earned. We cannot earn healing by living righteously. Unrighteous living cannot disqualify us for healing either. Healing is available for all because of Christ's sacrifice at the cross, no matter what their previous lifestyle has been. Repentance and the reception of forgiveness will often cleanse the conscience of one that has abused their body and allow them to receive healing as well.

You say that God wants people well. What about a sickness leading to death?

This common religious phrase *sickness leading to death* comes from misquoting a verse in the Gospel of John. Here is the verse:

> *But when Jesus heard it, He said, "This sickness is not unto death, but for the glory of God, that the Son of God may be glorified by it." John 11:4*

The verse actually says *this sickness is not unto death*. Christ is saying that Lazarus was not going to ultimately die from this sickness. He raised Lazarus from the dead.

Christ was not saying that some people are destined by God to die by sickness.

Death will eventually come to every man and woman who lives long enough. However, death can come without sickness or disability being involved. One can die in their sleep. One can lie down in health in their home and wake up in heaven. Sickness, injury and disability are not prerequisites for death. Death comes to the completely healthy also.

While many believers may die from sickness, this is not proof that God wanted to use sickness to bring them to heaven. Healing and health were available in Christ whether they received before their deaths. After the death of a believer, it is certain that they will receive what Christ has provided. The resurrection of believers will also be an eternal healing of their physical bodies. It is simply unfortunate for them and their loved ones that they did not receive healing before their deaths, but it is not tragic in an eternal sense for a believer to die by sickness.

What about curses, unforgiveness and other issues that seem to affect healing?

The Holy Spirit may supernaturally reveal other issues that prevent the reception of the grace of Christ in healing. However, it has been our experience that when faith in Christ as Healer is taught and doubts scripturally assaulted and destroyed that the vast majority of people can be healed. If we place emphasis where Christ placed emphasis, then our results will be more Christ-like in healing. Christ frequently taught about faith and doubt in reference to healing. He also taught about unforgiveness several times in His general teaching. On one occasion, He taught about curses. Therefore, we think that faith is the primary issue but other matters may also occasionally play a part. In the atmosphere of faith in Christ, the Holy Spirit often deals quickly with these other matters by a word of knowledge or discernment. Sometimes a "counseling session" may be required to get to the heart of the problem. Sometimes people who quickly lose their healing need this additional kind of ministry. They need to deal with the faith issues but may have another issue to deal with that blocks God's grace to them.

On rare occasions, a season of ministry may be necessary to resolve various issues in a few peoples' lives. For instance, with a few sick people there is hidden desire to remain sick because of laziness, irresponsibility or the desire to control through sickness. These people will outwardly present to everyone that they want to be well. Inwardly, however, they will have mixed motivations and will understand that being sick has its advantages. Until the hidden desire to be sick is repented of, no healing can take place. These people are often skilled at manipulation and fool practically everyone, even themselves, since their sickness is very real. These unfortunate people often get worse until the sickness is more than they can bear and then they repent of wanting to be sick. They often require a great deal of deliverance ministry and teaching in order for them to stay well. In our experience, these people probably are no more than one in a hundred Christians. They require compassionate confrontation and very patient ministry.

If God wants everyone healed, why does He need human beings to accomplish this?

God does supernaturally heal people without another human being involved. However, biblically it is clear that God much more often uses human beings to heal. The question above is probably best answered by posing a similar question. *If God wants everyone saved, why does He need human beings to accomplish this?* The answer is not easy but obviously involves

God maintaining the *free-will of human beings*. God could openly reveal Himself, override our wills and save and heal everyone. However, if God were to use this forceful means beyond the testimony, preaching and prayer of human beings, then human beings would not be able to freely choose to believe. They would believe because there would be no other choice. Faith, hope and love would no longer be the central and ultimate values of the universe but would be replaced by abject terror of God and servitude to avoid the consequences of not serving Him. God, our Father, has no wish for humanity to relate to Him in this manner. Quite the contrary, the Father wants people to love Him and to be loved by Him through Jesus Christ. Therefore, God has limited Himself by working through human beings.

Is there a "rule of thumb" to help determine what is the will of God in matters where someone is suffering?

Yes. There is a significant principle (beyond Christ's own example) that He revealed that can be used as a *rule of thumb*. Christ in Matthew 7:11 said:

> *If you then, being evil, know how to give good gifts to your children, how much more shall your Father who is in Heaven give what is good to those who ask Him.*

Christ is inviting us to compare what a normal parent would want for their children with what the Father wants for us. Christ is telling us that our common sense about what is good or bad is reliable in spiritual matters. In other words, if we would not do something harmful or bad to our own children, then the Father will not do it to us either. This principle cuts through complex theological thought that confuses good with evil. If common sense says the circumstance is bad, then our Father is not doing it to us. The Father will save, heal and deliver us through Christ.

Bibliography

Bauer, Walter, *A Greek-English Lexicon of New Testament and Other Early Christian Literatur*e, Second Edition, University of Chicago Press, Chicago, IL, 60637, 1979.

Sapp, Roger, *The Last Apostles on Earth*, All Nations Publications, P.O. Box 92847, Southlake, TX, 76092, 1995.

Vine, W.E., *The Expanded Vine's Expository Dictionary of New Testament Words*, Minneapolis, Minnesota; Bethany House Publishers, 1984.

Appendix A:
General (Mass) Healing Events
in the Synoptic Gospels

Mass Events	How Many Healed?	Size of Group?	Some Not Healed?
Event 1: Mt. 4:23-24	All is implied. *"every kind of disease and every kind of sickness"... "He healed them."*	Implied many. *"all the cities... news about Him went out into all Syria...all that were ill..."*	No. Strongly implied that all were healed since *"every kind"* were healed.
Event 2: Mt. 8:16-17	All is stated. *"healed all who were ill"*	*"many"*	No. *"all"* were healed who came to Christ.
Event 3: Mt. 9:35	All implied. *"every kind of disease & ... sickness"*	Implied many. *"all the cities"*	No. Implies all were healed since *"every kind"* were healed.
Event 4: Mt.15:30-31	All is implied. *"...He healed them.."*	*"great multitudes"*	No. No mention of any one not healed.
Event 5: Mk.1:32-34	Many is stated. *"many"*	Implied many. *"the whole city"*	None mentioned. Verses do not allow absolute clarity.
Event 6: Mk. 3:9-11	*"many"*	*"the multitude"*	None mentioned. Verses do not allow absolute clarity.
Event 7: Mk. 6:2-6	*"Few"*: *"He could do no miracle there except that He laid His hands on a few sick people and healed them"*	Only a small number of people is implied. Not many came to Him for healing apparently.	Strongly implied that some could have been healed that were not because of their unbelief in Christ.
Event 8: Lk. 4:40	All is implied. *"...He was healing them."*	All is implied. *"all who had any sick... brought them.."*	No. Passage implies that all were healed.
Event 9: Lk. 5:15-16	All is implied.	*"great multitudes"*	No. Passage implies that all were healed.
Event 10: Lk. 6:17-19	*"all"*	*"a great multitude... a great throng..."*	No. *"healing them all"*
Event 11: Lk. 9:11	All is implied.	*"multitudes"*	No. Implies that needy were healed.

Appendix B
25 Individual Healings in Christ's Ministry

Description	Matthew	Mark	Luke	John
Blindness Healed				
Two Blind Men	9:27-31			
Bethsaida's Blind Man		8:22-26		
Man Born Blind				9:1-41
Blind Bartimaeus	20:29-34	10:46-52	18:35-43	
**Blind & Mute Man	12:22-24			
Healing of Conditions Caused by Demons				
Demoniac Boy	17:14-21	9:14-29	9:37-43a	
Gaderene Demoniac	8:28-34	5:1-20	8:26-27	
*Mute Demoniac	9:32-35		11:14-15	
**Blind & Mute Man	12:22-24			
Woman's Daughter	15:21-28	7:24-30		
Nobleman's Son				4:46-54
Healing of the Deaf and Mute				
Deaf/Mute in Decapolis		7:31-37		
*Mute Demoniac	9:32-35		11:14-15	
The Cleansing of Lepers				
Leper	8:1-4	1:40-45	5:12-16	
Ten Lepers			17:11-19	
Resurrections				
Lazarus Raised				11:1-46
Widow's Son Raised			7:11-18	
Jairus' Daughter Raised	9:18-26	5:21-43	8:40-56	
Healing of Physical Disabilities & Injuries				
Imfirmed Man				5:1-9
Paralytic Man & Friends	9:1-8	2:1-12	5:17-26	
Man's Withered Hand	12:9-13	3:1-7a	6:6-11	
Crippled Woman			13:10-17	
Man with Dropsy			14:1-6	
***Malchus' Ear	26:51	14:47	22:51	18:10
Healing of Sickness or Conditions				
Centurion's Servant	8:5-13		7:1-10	
Woman's Issue of Blood	9:20-22	5:25-34	8:43-48	
Peter's Mother in Law	8:14-15	1:29-31	4:38-39	

*Chart repeats this healing in two categories.

**Chart repeats this healing in two categories.

*** Only Luke reveals that Christ healed the ear that had been cut off.

Available from the author:
The Last Apostles on Earth,
Modern Apostles and Apostolic Ministry, 186 pages, 1995. $10.00
Order from All Nations Publications 1-817-514-0653

"The 1990's is a decade characterized by the rise of the modern day apostolic movement. *The Last Apostles on Earth* is, therefore, very timely. It provides us with valuable biblical information for building a theological framework within to understand this work of the Holy Spirit in our day." *Dr. C. Peter Wagner, Fuller Seminary*

"*The Last Apostles on Earth* is a fresh and unique look at what Scripture says about apostolic ministry. This book is a must read for anyone wanting to account for the biblical evidence regarding apostles in the Church today." *Dr. Gary Greig, Professor, Regent Univ. School of Theology*

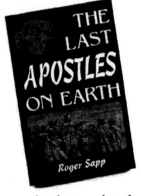

Ministries Today Magazine Review: "If you thought the latest wave of revival manifestations stirred up the church, wait until the next one crests! The author of this new book says that the next big revival wave will bring genuine apostolic ministry to the surface. Dr. Roger Sapp believes that in the latter part of the 1990's, Christ will freshly call, restore and anoint apostles as gift ministries to the church. This author writes in order to prepare local leaders to relate to these mobile ministers, and he explores and applies biblical principles about apostles. Roger Sapp, (formerly) a theology teacher at a Virginia college, explores Old Testament kings as types of New Testament apostles. That analogy, though limited, helps show how apostles conduct the affairs of the Kingdom of God. Many insights await any careful reader... This book does not simply study apostles as a topic. Apostles come alive as real people sent from God and as the Lord's final thrust to bring the Church age to a glorious close. If the church is to obey the Great Commission before Jesus returns, the author contends, we will need to end with even greater power than the first apostles displayed. As end-time revival waves break upon humanity, this book urges us to grab our surfboards and prepare for the last great ride of church history: the whole church reaching the whole world with the whole gospel. "

"I really appreciate Roger Sapp's approach to this important subject. He seeks to arrive at a biblical answer in the face of an emotionally charged environment. You may not agree, but you'll face some real questions head on". Dudley Hall, President, Successful Christian Living Ministries

What does the Bible teach concerning women in ministry? Is there a difference between men and women in roles in the Church? Is "equality" in the Church taught by the Bible? Is there a biblical reason to make exceptions for the normal "rules" for certain women?

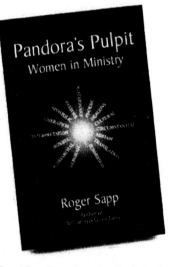

Pandora's Pulpit answers these questions and many others candidly and courageously. It exposes the extremes presently being taught and practiced in the Church. *Pandora's Pulpit* is destined to become a classic on the role of women in the present renewal.

Pandora's Pulpit offers a summary of various modern attempts to reject the New Testament's basic teaching concerning women and their role in the Church. It reveals the divine reasons why the New Testament teaches what it does about women's ministries. Most importantly this book describes the predictable outcomes of teaching disobedience to these important New Testament truths in the lives of women, men and their children.

Controversial title? Let us explain. In early 1998, Roger Sapp heard messages from prominent leaders and read four recent and popular charismatic books that were teaching a unkind and false doctrine about modern apostles and discipling others. As a result, he has written a courageous and pointed book that addresses the following questions: What does the Bible teach concerning modern apostolic fathers and their relationships with other Christians? Do these ministry

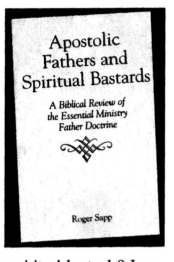

Apostolic
Fathers and
Spiritual Bastards

A Biblical Review of
the Essential Ministry
Father Doctrine

Roger Sapp

fathers save spiritual sons from being spiritual bastards? Is an intimate relationship with a ministry father essential to please God? Are ministries inherited from ministry fathers? Do all properly prepared ministries become ministry fathers? Is the true foundation of spiritual inheritance in the Kingdom of God the relationships between fathers and sons? What does the apostle Paul's phrase *you have not many fathers* really mean? In this new book, Roger Sapp answers these questions and many others as he confronts this very popular heresy head on. He compares with Scripture and with insight analyzes this unkind and unscriptural teaching that unfairly marks some Christians as *spiritual bastards* or orphans. He calls the Church back to a balanced and scriptural approach to apostolic ministry and the discipleship of others. Every leader needs to read this courageous and pointed book! This book is subtitled *A Biblical Review of the Essential Ministry Father Doctrine.* It is 110 pages and includes the popular *Honoring the Truth-teller* articles as an appendix.

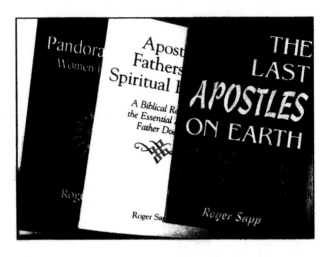
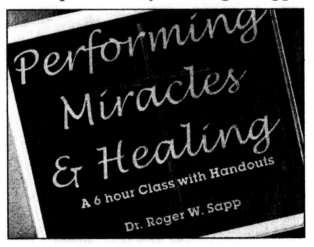

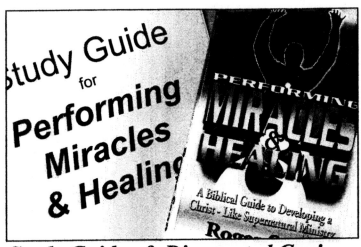

Study Guides & Discounted Copies of Performing Miracles & Healing (PMH)

Study Guides contain 1130 questions in 162 pages in 8 ½" x 11" book form. Certificates available on completion of course contained in Study Guide.

1 Study Guide (*without PMH or Answer Guide*) $15 plus $4 shipping

1 Study and 1 Answer Guide (*without PMH*) $30 plus $4 shipping

Group Study Assortment #1: 5 Study Guides, 5 copies PMH,
1 Answer Guide $160 (includes $10 shipping, 10% discount)
Group Study Assortment #2: 10 Study Guides, 10 copies of PMN,
1 Answer Guide $300 (includes $20 shipping, 20% discount)
Group Study Assortment #3: 20 Study Guides, 20 copies of PMH,
1 Answer Guide $460 (includes $30 shipping, 30% discount)

Single copies of PMH: $19 (includes $4 shipping)
2 copies of PMH: $34 (includes $4 shipping)
3 copies of PMH: $49 (includes $4 shipping)
5 copies of PMH: $73 (includes $6 ship. & 10% discount)
10 copies of PMH: $130 (includes $10 ship. & 20% discount)
20 copies of PMH: $230 (includes $20 ship. & 30% discount)
30 copies (1 case) PMH: $300 (incl. $30 ship, 40% discount)

Call 1-817-514-0653 for credit card orders or mail check to
All Nations Publications, P.O. Box 92847, Southlake, Texas 76092